Learning Therapeutic Storytelling

AF172750

Stefan Hammel

Learning Therapeutic Storytelling

The Essentials at a Glance

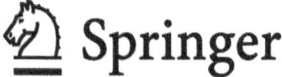 Springer

Stefan Hammel
Institut für Hypnosystemische
Beratung
Kaiserslautern, Germany

ISBN 978-3-662-69109-0   ISBN 978-3-662-69110-6   (eBook)
https://doi.org/10.1007/978-3-662-69110-6

Translation from the German language edition: "Therapeutisches Erzählen lernen"
by Stefan Hammel, © The Editor(s) and The Author(s), under exclusive license to
Springer-Verlag GmbH, DE, part of Springer Nature 2023. Published by Springer
Berlin Heidelberg. All Rights Reserved.

This book is a translation of the original German edition "Therapeutisches Erzählen
lernen" by Stefan Hammel, published by Springer-Verlag GmbH, DE in 2023. The
translation was done with the help of an artificial intelligence machine translation
tool. A subsequent human revision was done primarily in terms of content, so that
the book will read stylistically differently from a conventional translation. Springer
Nature works continuously to further the development of tools for the production
of books and on the related technologies to support the authors.

This Springer imprint is published by the registered company Springer-Verlag
GmbH, DE, part of Springer Nature.
The registered company address is: Heidelberger Platz 3, 14197 Berlin, Germany

If disposing of this product, please recycle the paper.

Preface: I'd Rather do it Right Away!—Can You Learn That Quickly too?

Can one learn to tell stories? Without a doubt, this is possible, because like everything in the world, stories have a structure that can be described and therefore taught. It's no coincidence that there are writing schools for authors, courses for fairy tale tellers, and the like. But what about stories that are told in therapy, stories that have a strengthening, building, healing effect? Something like the wisdom stories from earlier times. Perhaps not for all people at the same time, but for the person who is sitting across from you... Would such a thing be possible? Are there such things as therapeutic stories? If so, how do you recognize them? How are they structured? How do they work? Their use and their effect should also follow some rules that can be learned and taught.

This book is dedicated to people who do not want to wait to tell healing stories until perhaps, with some luck, old age wisdom comes, but who would rather start right away, so to speak, right now—well aware that this is also a field in which one can learn new things for a long time and refine the skills already acquired.

It is dedicated to those who do not want to leave the telling of therapeutic stories to a happy inspiration (which is certainly also welcome), but want to understand the rules this storytelling follows, how to develop new therapeutic stories at any time in a conversation or recognize proven stories as relevant for this situation and tell them effectively.

The desire to want to learn something big in a short time seems legitimate to me considering the many things there are to learn and discover in the world.

I firmly believe that one can achieve quite a lot with relatively little effort in the field of therapeutic storytelling, to put it mildly—of course, mastery requires more. However, it seems to me that there is little guidance available so far. While there is a lot of literature with stories that could be used in therapy, there is little on how such stories can be individually developed and adapted to the needs of each client. Even the question of how we know how to appropriately assign stories that we encounter in therapeutic literature to the life stories that clients tell us, so that they have a good effect, is often left unanswered. I have already attempted to fill this gap once, fifteen years ago. While the "Handbook of Therapeutic Storytelling" (Hammel 2018) that I wrote then takes an extensive look at the healing effect of stories, this book is primarily aimed at people who want to use the little time they have for reading and learning in a particularly focused way. In a small space, it conveys when and how stories become therapeutically effective and, despite its brevity, regularly delves into the illustrative, into the telling of therapeutic stories. The goal is thus to feed both halves of the brain. While the left half is said to be good at dealing with rules and structure, it corresponds to the wisdom of the right half when we say: You learn storytelling by telling stories.

As a background to the therapeutic storytelling presented here, it is first necessary to refer to the work of the American hypnotherapy pioneer Milton Erickson. Erickson regularly embedded his suggestions in stories. At least three quarters of his therapeutic work was carried out without trance inductions or hypnotic trance states in the classical sense (Schmidt 2004, p. 69), but rather in a more awake dialogue with clients, one could say, in a conversational trance. To illustrate a point that seemed important to him, Erickson told his patients and training candidates anecdotes from his own life, experiences and case examples from his work, success and failure stories from the world of sports, childhood memories, family experiences, and much more. One goal he pursued with these stories was to induce a questioning, curious, searching, and learning attitude in his listeners, thus preparing the ground for an impending change. Erickson was of the opinion that unconscious areas of experience, which can be addressed by stories, are much more suitable for developing solutions than the conscious understanding of problem dynamics and causes. For him, stories were a way to stimulate the unconscious to find solutions (Rosen 1982).

Another great storyteller who has influenced the concepts presented here in the background is the Austrian psychologist, philosopher, and communication researcher Paul Watzlawick, a valued friend and companion of Erickson's. Watzlawick once mentioned that he primarily speaks and writes in stories because he can only think in stories. Everything that is not pictorial is difficult for him to grasp. Similar to Erickson, Watzlawick uses examples from diverse research and life areas to illustrate structures of successful and unsuccessful communication in such a way that the reader can involuntarily apply them to his situation or pass them on to other people (Watzlawick 1976, 1983; Watzlawick et al 2011).

The work of Erickson, Watzlawick, and their colleagues led to the development of Systemic Therapy with centers in Palo Alto (California), Milan, and Heidelberg, and the hypnosystemic therapy following the Heidelberg physician and therapist Gunther Schmidt. The systemic and hypnosystemic traditions have significantly influenced therapeutic storytelling. At first glance, this influence may seem less apparent than that of the two great storytellers Erickson and Watzlawick, but in the background, the concepts of systemic therapy are important for the presented narrative style. Mention should be made here of the importance of appreciative connotation, reframing, circular causality, the self-stabilization of systems, the orientation of therapy towards resources, relationships, goals, and desires of clients within the framework of systemic work. Hypnosystemic work shapes therapeutic storytelling by addressing involuntary processes instead of conscious thinking. Goals that the client cannot consciously achieve can still be pursued because his body or unconscious instances can probably implement them, even if the client cannot explain how this happens. Characteristic of hypnosystemic work is also the inclusion of concepts from psychodrama, structural constellations, and part concepts, which divide the individual into a group of partial personalities or personality aspects. The division of individuality (which literally means "indivisibility") into an "inner parliament", "inner team", an "inner family" or similar is reflected in many stories in which ambivalent experiences are distributed among various protagonists, landscape elements, functions of a thing, attempts at a solution by a character, etc. (Hammel 2018, 253 ff., 2011, 259, 159, 2014, 206 ff., 2022, 145 ff.)

Another influence arises from the Jewish-Christian, Oriental, and particularly biblical narrative tradition. The stories that Jesus told aim to convey content in the form of example stories and metaphors (or, more accurately, parables) that can be useful for social, psychological, and spiritual orientation in the world. The same applies to many other stories in the tradition of the Old and New Testaments (Bible according to Martin Luther 2016), in the later Jewish (Bonder 2021; Eliach 1997) and Christian tradition (Bukowski 1994; Domanski 2022) and the Oriental (Aceval 2015; Schami 1987) narrative art.

Stefan Hammel

References

Aceval C (2015) Der Mann, der nicht sterben wollte. Märchen aus dem Maghreb. Papermoon, Schönaich

Bibel nach Martin Luthers Übersetzung (2016) Standardausgabe. Ohne Apokryphen. Bibelgesellschaft, Stuttgart

Bonder N (2021) Der Rabbi hat immer recht. Die Kunst, Probleme zu lösen. Carl Auer, Heidelberg

Bukowski P (1994) Die Bibel ins Gespräch bringen. Erwägungen zu einer Grundfrage der Seelsorge. Vandenhoeck, Göttingen

Domanski J (2022) Worte, die wirken. Einführung in die hypnosystemische Seelsorge. Gütersloher, Gütersloh

Eliach Y (1997) Träume vom Überleben. Chassidische Geschichten aus dem 20. Jahrhundert. Herder, Freiburg

Hammel S (2006) Der Grashalm in der Wüste. Metaphern und Geschichten in Beratung, Therapie und Seelsorge. impress, Mainz

Hammel S (2009) Handbuch des therapeutischen Erzählens. Geschichten und Metaphern in Psychotherapie, Kinder- und Familientherapie, Heilkunde, Coaching und Supervision. Klett-Cotta, Stuttgart

Hammel S (2012) The blade of grass in the desert. Storytelling: Forgotten medicine for healing the soul. A story of 100 stories for counselling and therapy. impress, Mainz

Hammel S (2016) Loslassen und Leben. Befreiende Geschichten. impress, Mainz

Hammel S (2018) Handbook of therapeutic storytelling. Stories and metaphors in psychotherapy, child and family therapy, medical treatment, coaching and supervision. Routledge, London

Rosen S (Hrsg) (2009) Die Lehrgeschichten von Milton H. Erickson. Iskopress, Salzhausen

Schami R (1987) Das letzte Wort der Wanderratte. Märchen, Fabeln und phantastische Geschichten. dtv, München

Schmidt G (2004) Liebesaffären zwischen Problem und Lösung. Hypnosystemisches Arbeiten in schwierigen Kontexten. Carl Auer, Heidelberg

Watzlawick P (1978) Wie wirklich ist die Wirklichkeit? Wahn, Täuschung, Verstehen. Piper, München

Watzlawick P (1988) Anleitung zum Unglücklichsein. Piper, München

Watzlawick P, et al (1974) Lösungen. Zur Theorie und Praxis menschlichen Wandels

Contents

About the Author

Stefan Hammel works as a systemic therapist, hypnotherapist, and author, as a Protestant hospital and psychiatric chaplain, as well as the head of the Institute for Hypnosystemic Counseling in Kaiserslautern and as a speaker of systemic and hypnotherapeutic training institutes in Germany, Austria, and Switzerland. He conducts seminars on Ericksonian hypnotherapy, therapeutic storytelling, systemic and hypnosystemic counseling. His main areas of work are in couple and family therapy, child and adolescent therapy, depression, anxiety, trauma, end-of-life and grief counseling, as well as the support of somatic healing.

1

What does Storytelling Have to do With Therapy?—Life as a Story

Trailer

People tell stories and stories shape our experiences. Dreams are stories, older than verbal language, a kind of mother tongue of the soul. They encounter us as a mixture of memory, expectation, and imagination. They allow us to try out options for action and test possibilities of experience without endangering our lives or our position in a group. They can re-regulate our reactions to experiences and thus bring us back from overwhelming experiences to the ability to act. Psychotherapy can use this circumstance to dissolve burdensome stories and develop stories that expand possibilities.

Every day we tell ourselves stories, about failed or successful, threatened and saved lives. What if not only life produces our stories, but also the stories generate our life and experiences? Then retelling our life stories might be the redesign of our lives!

© The Author(s), under exclusive license to Springer-Verlag GmbH, DE, part of Springer Nature 2024
S. Hammel, *Learning Therapeutic Storytelling*,
https://doi.org/10.1007/978-3-662-69110-6_1

If one understands life as a stream of stories that we tell ourselves and each other, then psychotherapy might also be the dissolution and transformation of restrictive stories and the development and stabilization of stories that expand possibilities.

Therapeutic Stories as Healing Dreams

Anyone who watches a pet sleep can sometimes make an interesting observation. A dog, for example, will sometimes growl or bark softly in its sleep, run around with rapidly moving paws while lying in its place, prick up its ears or excitedly wag its tail. It looks as if he is involved in a fight—perhaps he is chasing another animal or he has to deal with a rival. The situation hardly allows any other conclusion than that the animal is dreaming in moving scenes.

Our day and night dreams are stories, a kind of stories that are older than human language and much older than humanity itself. They could be referred to—along with communication in emotions and body reactions—as the mother tongue of the soul.

One difference between night and day dreams is that day dreams react immediately to new impulses, while night dreams usually process the experiences of the previous day. Due to the low density of new stimuli at night, they can deal with the current situation in greater thoroughness and depth.

In terms of content, night dreams often deal with experiences that could not be adequately processed during the day—because of their intensity, external distraction, or a desire for self-distraction to avoid painful thoughts. It can be noted that night dreams often have a metaphorical character, while day dreams tend to realistically depict experienced or potentially experienceable situations. Otherwise, as far as I can see, there is no fundamental difference between the two.

One advantage of dreams (in sleep as well as in wakefulness) is that our dream consciousness, which could also be called subconscious or unconscious, can try out options for action in a highly realistic way, with all senses and emotions. What proves successful leads to feelings of happiness, associated with an involuntarily understood invitation: "Do what corresponds to this dream!". What does not prove successful leads to fear, horror, anger, and sadness, associated with the implicit warning: "Avoid what corresponds to this dream!" Above all, however, our possibilities for action and experience can be tried out safely in the dream, i.e., without the risk of endangering our health, our life, our position in a group, and our belonging to it.

What might a dog dream when it twitches its paws, tail, and ears in its sleep? He could dream of how he attacks the hated big neighbor's dog from a hiding place and bites into his fur. They would roll across the street as a hissing ball, until in the end—but the neighbor's dog wins. Our dog wakes up and knows what he'd better not try.

Apart from looking ahead at possible future experiences and evaluating their significance for the individual and group, dreams can also be useful for evaluating past events in terms of their significance for the dreamer and his social environment. In dreams that process past events, it is often about re-regulating strong feelings such as loneliness, fear, anger, or sadness and associated body reactions such as agitation or rigidity, in order to bring a person back from overwhelming experiences to a state of high ability to act.

One goal of dreams can be to bring people out of states of passive suffering, of ignoring dangers or of diffuse hyperreactivity into a regulated experience and behavior in which they take control of and shape their lives.

Our dreams are stories, and our stories are dreams. Not all of these stories are of a fictional nature. Also our memories and expectations, which we hold for our past and future, have the shape of stories that we dream again and again in a similar way and sometimes completely new.

No boundary can be drawn between our dreams as a supposed unreality and a "real reality". Paul Watzlawick has dedicated an entire book to the topic: "How Real is Real? Confusion, Disinformation, Communication" (Watzlawick 1976). This means, "Reality consists of nothing else but stories" (Schlippe and Schweitzer 1996, p. 40) and "our inner images create our realities" (Groß and Popper 2020, p. 76).

How Reality and Fiction Blend and Become One
Memory dreams and fictional dreams—as stories of what our past could have been—often mix in wild succession, until we sometimes no longer know what was originally memory and what was fiction, or until we mistake one for the other. Our expectation dreams, however, no matter how realistic we may consider them, are always fictional, because no one has visited the future and could testify to things that are yet to happen.

We dream the present (unless we want to divide it into a recent past and an imminent future) in the form of interpreted perception—whereby any connection we assert with "if" and "then", with "because", "therefore" and "for", has already left the realm of a neutral description of mere facts.

On the way home from a team meeting, for example, I could remember how a colleague made an ironic remark about the quality of my work in front of the whole team. "You jerk!" I would remember that I didn't say it, but thought it, and how I was initially too stunned to respond, how I then just said he should stop the bullying and he replied that he could gladly put facts on the table to back up his claims if I thought this was about bullying. I could remember how I actually wanted to say: "You would even shoot people to get ahead!", but then left the room wordlessly with a lump in my throat. The next scene I imagine could be me telling my partner at home what happened. In the process, I add sarcastic comments about the colleague to the narrative of the event. I'm still upset that I was too surprised to react well. Therefore, I imagine the scene with a good response that surprises the colleague. I imagine how he reacts, how I respond again, and how the team members react. Then I think of an even better response to the colleague and play through the scene with it. Next, I consider how I will be prepared for the next team meeting. What can I say to get back at him or what remarks can I keep in reserve that fit as universally as possible to all his meanness? When I later tell my partner about the team meeting, I have already played through so many variations of the event that I am no longer sure what exactly the colleague said and what I actually responded.

In the cinema of the mind, what is associated with each other often mixes until the actual and fictional events, facts and interpretations can hardly be distinguished. Thus, actual memories, fictional memories, expectable and unlikely future events, interpretations of the intentions and character assessments of other people, presentation of facts and assessments of future perspectives merge. We tell ourselves stories by looking and listening inwardly at what we have experienced, while we shorten parts of the event, add parts and sometimes significantly alter the event. People call the results of such processes "reality".

Reality is What we Call Reality
Watzlawick, Weakland, and Fish summarize this by saying that "reality is what we have come to call 'reality'." (Watzlawick et al. 2011, p. 130). Von Schlippe and Schweitzer write that what we call "reality" arises in

dialogue, in other words, what we consider as "real" is learned in a lengthy process of socialization and verbalization within a society or group. Realities are therefore a construct of systems that have reached a consensus on how things should be seen. This shared view of a society is significantly determining when people experience themselves as satisfied ("happy") or dissatisfied ("unhappy") (Schlippe and Schweitzer 1996, p. 89).

Reality-creating dialogues range from one-on-one conversations to the broad societal discourse of a tradition spanning millennia. These dialogues create collective realities that people join and inadvertently constitute a "we" with all others who identify with the same reality construction. Likewise, internal dialogues create individual realities that we shape in self-talk and daydreams and that develop unnoticed, slowly and steadily, like dunes moving as waves through the desert, so we do not perceive the change in the landscape. Thus, from the external striving for belonging and agreement and the internal striving for identity and integrity, personal realities emerge that we believe in and by which we orient ourselves.

If the reality of human experience is now something other than facticity—which reality or what image of reality is then the basis for therapy? Watzlawick explains with regard to psychotherapy, if it is true that reality is always a constructed one, it is about replacing a person's suffering, no longer viable reality construction with another, more viable one. (Maurer 2021)

In the same tradition, Elvira Muffler explains that hypnosystemic therapy provides "support in changing the construction of *reality* (as that which *works* in people)." (Muffler 2015, p. 21)

From this perspective, it might be beneficial if we reframe the painful, so-called reality of clients with additional stories that they experience as plausible. It is not so important whether they view our stories as "reality" or as "fiction". For the world of their inner films, any narrated reality or fiction can be a relevant contribution to the memories, interpretations, and expectations that they view as the original story of their life. The only important thing is that the physiology, the world of emotions and physical reactions of the clients, responds helpfully when new perspectives arise from listening, which expand the frame of interpretation and action possibilities for them. Then they come into an experience of regulated feeling and mobility instead of rigidity, numbness, or emotional overload, i.e., into a state in which they shape their situations instead of suffering them.

The Plasticity of Memories

To further illustrate the plasticity of memories, I would like to give an example. A woman reports in therapy the following: When she leaves home, she checks twenty to thirty times whether the stove is turned off. If the stove is not turned off, there could be a fire. This could burn down the house and neighbors could die. In that case, it would be her fault. I ask why it is not enough to check the stove once. She explains that after she has left the kitchen, she checks again in her mind whether she really checked the stove. To do this, she recalls her memory of it. Because she really wants to be 100 percent sure not to be at fault, she wonders whether she knows for sure that this is the memory of just now or whether it could also be the memory of yesterday or the day before. If there is no evidence that it is today's memory, she checks the stove again. Of course, she has learned to mention the current date when checking. But while she remembers in front of the kitchen how she said the date, she wonders: "Am I absolutely sure that I said: 'Today is February 8th' or could it also be that I said: 'Today is February 7th'?" If she is not sure, she checks the stove again. When she checks outside the kitchen again whether her memory tells her that she has turned off the stove and sees the image of it in her mind's eye, she wonders: Is this a real memory or could it also be a mere imagination? To test this, she produces an inner image of what the stove would look like if the stove was still on, and she asks herself: Which image is more intense: The one from the presumed memory or the one from the presumed fiction? Once she has made a decision, she wonders whether she is sure that the image from the presumed fiction was actually weaker than the one from the presumed memory. If she is not sure, she repeats the test several times. In the process, the fictitious inner image of the switched-on stove becomes more vivid and emotionally intense. Is she still sure now which image is a memory and which is just a comparison image for testing purposes? If she is not sure, she checks the stove again…

This is necessary because in between she regularly sees the burning house, the neighbor being carried out dying on a stretcher or charred by the fire brigade, and the judge asking her if she did not check the stove.

Perception, factual and value judgments, actual and fictitious memories with different versions of a possible future merge into each other here as well. Our daydreams are shaped by memories and expectations and merge experienced and fictitious content into an experienced reality. In the eyes of others, these dreams may seem close to reality, far from reality, or entirely fictitious. The transitions between these categories are fluid.

Language as a Coding System for Stories
In order for such dreams to become told and heard stories, language is needed. Language can be understood as a coding system through which our dreams have become communicable, so that other people can decode the stories

that we generate within us and also see, feel and hear them within themselves. If these people identify with us, i.e., involuntarily sympathize, they will probably also show similar emotions and other physiological reactions as we experience them while imagining and telling.

Stories that are told over and over again in a group can increase the cohesion in a group. They can also distinguish this group from other groups. They can assign a certain role to individual members in the group and ensure that the group members behave according to the rules of the group. If the group members can agree in the form of told stories on who in the group has which role and what he is therefore allowed or not allowed to do, this may possibly contribute to the fact that this question does not have to be settled with weapons or fists. However, it can also mean that words have become weapons in this group, and it is not excluded that the use of words is followed by the use of weapons.

Stories as Offers of Roles and Identity

The stories we tell ourselves can serve to assign roles to ourselves and especially to each other: It seems to me that the roles we assign to ourselves through stories, if they remain unchallenged, become our identity. The same applies if the contradiction to such a role and identity assignment cannot assert itself in the group and in the individual because it is met with violence and the individual cannot withdraw from the group on which it depends.

This is experienced, for example, by children who have to accept the humiliations of their parents and siblings because any resistance leads to even more severe humiliations. They must accept the role assignment conveyed in this way and the accompanying binding offer of identity because they are not offered an alternative location in the system and not having a place in the family system or leaving the system is not a viable option for them.

In a certain way, the situation is similar for people in an organization or a closed institution (boarding school, barracks, prison, closed psychiatry) when all (or most or the dominant) members of the system treat them as sick or inferior. If they manage not to develop an unfavorable identity experience from the stressful role assignment, it is because people from their past (such as the family of origin) or in a special function (such as the therapist, social worker or chaplain) have made them a plausible, alternative offer of their identity, which is vivid to them and which they experience as present. (For this struggle between two competing identities, see the poem "Who am I?", which Dietrich Bonhoeffer wrote in his imprisonment (http://www.dbonhoeffer.org/who-was-db2.htm)).

Not only individually told stories, but also the stories of a group about its members and individuals or groups outside the narrative of the "good ones", who distinguish themselves as "we" from others, have a potential to burden and traumatize people. Stories with a potential to hurt are often those with which people depict others as inferior or not equal. Often it is about the demarcation of territories in a broader sense: What am I allowed to do and what are you allowed to do? Who is right? Who is to blame? Who do you choose—her or me? What do you choose—the family or your own path?

References

Groß M, Popper V (2020) Und die Maus hört ein Rauschen. Hypnosystemisches Erleben in Therapie, Coaching und Beratung. (Reden reicht nicht?!) Carl Auer, Heidelberg

Maurer A (2021) Radiokolleg, Teil 4. Der optimistische Nihilist Paul Watzlawick. ORF-broadcast of 29.7.21

Muffler E (ed) (2015) Kommunikation in der Psychoonkologie. Ein hypnosystemischer Ansatz. Carl Auer, Heidelberg

Von Schlippe A, Schweitzer J (1996) Lehrbuch der systemischen Beratung. Vandenhoeck, Göttingen

Watzlawick P (1976) How Real is Real? Confusion, Disinformation, Communication. Norton, New York

Watzlawick, P et al (2011) Change. Principles of Problem Formation and Problem Resolution. Norton, New York

2

When is Storytelling Therapeutic?—Hurtful and Healing Stories

Trailer

This chapter is about when stories can be hurtful or healing. The latter occurs when it is possible to transform or replace previously degrading, energy-consuming, possibility-limiting life stories into appreciative, energy-giving, possibility-expanding stories for the listener. The context in which a story is told is at least as important for its effect as the content. In therapy, stories are listened to with the expectation that they will contribute to a solution. The client's concern creates a framework in which the helpful aspects of the story gain more intense effectiveness than if it were read in a book, for example.

If stories can hurt, they can also heal. But when is a story therapeutically effective? Certainly, there are stories that prove themselves time and again in therapy and those that will rarely prove themselves in therapy. Nevertheless, it seems to me that the context in which the story is told,

© The Author(s), under exclusive license to Springer-Verlag
GmbH, DE, part of Springer Nature 2024
S. Hammel, *Learning Therapeutic Storytelling*,
https://doi.org/10.1007/978-3-662-69110-6_2

the "when", "where" and "how" of the telling, contributes at least as much to the therapeutic effectiveness as the content of the story—which is why this book presents therapeutically proven stories without claiming that a story is "always" or "never" therapeutically valuable.

Hurtful Stories

Every day we produce and reproduce a multitude of memory, expectation, and interpretation stories. Some of these are helpful by expanding our possibilities of thinking, acting, and self-experiencing and putting us in a position of actively shaping our lives. Others have unwanted side effects and are harmful overall, as they limit our thinking and action possibilities, drain our energy, and put us in a position of passive suffering or blind rage.

Of course, the stories we tell ourselves and each other every day and by which we align our lives also have far-reaching systemic effects.

For example, an employee might view the executives in his company as "social responsibility bearers" or as "capitalist pigs". Even if he never publicly labels them as such, his viewpoint will influence how his colleagues and superiors interact with him and ultimately with each other through unconscious processes.

Healing Stories

Stories have a therapeutic effect when they transform degrading, energy-consuming (demotivating), and possibility-limiting life stories into appreciative, energy-giving (motivating), and possibility-expanding stories—or when they replace stories of the first category with those of the second type in a way that is plausible for the clients. Here, "replacing" does not necessarily mean that the previously nurtured burdensome stories are somehow deleted. It is sufficient if important, framing narratives belong to the second category, so that appreciative and confident views dominate the interpretation of one's own life.

Therapeutic stories are healing dreams, i.e., those that do better for our self-image and worldview, our energy balance, our ability to act, and the happiness we experience than the stories we have previously told ourselves.

The Narrative Situation as Part of the Message

When I said that the "when", "where", and "how" of a story contribute at least as much to its effect as the content of the story itself, the discussion of these relationships should be worth a few more words. While we can certainly tell the same stories in a conversation among friends or in a therapy session, it makes a big difference in which context a story is told.

The setting of the therapy session contains a frame suggestion that determines the interpretation of all content communicated therein. Clients usually come to therapy to find help. Stories are listened to here with the expectation that they were selected by the therapist to contribute to a solution. Therefore, clients will involuntarily search everything presented to them here for its contribution to addressing their concern and will attribute special relevance to their personal life to what they discover on this search. The helpful aspects of the story thereby gain more intense effectiveness. The story is scanned for its therapeutic benefit due to the therapeutic context. If the client encounters the same story in an entertaining book, it takes on a different meaning: firstly, it is not told to them personally in their unique life situation, and secondly, it seems to be intended only for the reader's entertainment and not to influence their life circumstances. The story is then read with a view to its entertainment value and understood as part of an invented reality without a special reference to life. The story is, so to speak, scanned with a different initial question. This results in different feedback on its relevance to life. This means that a story changes its meaning with the context in which it is told.

Rescued Bumblebee

My parents had a swimming pool in the garden. My father was responsible for its regular cleaning. Once he found a bumblebee that was swimming in the water and struggling for its life. Very carefully, he slid his hand under it and lifted it out of the water. The bumblebee immediately stung him in the hand. "I didn't even know that bumblebees could sting. I was quite surprised!", said my father. But he was also annoyed and outraged. "You save such an animal and then it shows itself so ungrateful!", was his thought. "Actually, one should punish the bumblebee!" But he then came to a more merciful judgment. The bumblebee was given a place on the lawn, and the hand was treated with cooling ointment.

I could tell this parable to a foster mother who is worried because the child she has adopted rejects her love, or to staff in a child and adolescent psychiatry who suffer from physical attacks by their charges.

The story could be told to a man who laments that he has provided a good life for his young Eastern European, African, or Asian partner, and she has now left him for another man.

It could also be told to a patient who is struggling with his body after an allergic shock or another sudden health crisis.

The story can also be applied in other situations where people feel "abandoned".

With the therapeutic context, the spectrum of possible interpretations by the listener shifts each time.

The Recipient as Part of the Message

Not only when, where, and how we tell a story influences the meaning the story has, but also to *whom* we tell it.

An example: Together with some other authors, I have produced card sets with therapeutic stories—on one side an inspiring picture, on the other a matching story (Hammel et al. 2018 among others). Now there are therapists who let their clients choose a card by orienting themselves on the picture on the front. Then they read them the story on the back. Again and again, there are therapists who report back: "The story fit perfectly!" and clients who marvel and say: "This is exactly the story I need right now!" One might see behind this the guidance of an invisible power or a wise unconscious that clients draw exactly the "right" card. Personally, I suggest the view that possibly every potentially therapeutic story or at least a very large spectrum of such stories is made by the client's unconscious into "exactly the right" story in his situation by creatively linking the helpful aspects of the narrative with his situation. The therapist could therefore also draw any card from the stack before the session, announce to the client: "I think I have found exactly the right story for you and your situation. May I read it to you?" The probability that the client agrees: "Indeed!" because his unconscious makes "exactly the right" story out of this story, is quite high.

"It's like working with tarot cards or astrology—it works because something in the person working with it is set in motion," a seminar participant commented in this context. I responded to her with another image that illustrates how the conscious and the unconscious are two separate areas that can communicate with each other when they are meaningfully related.

Dowsers

Think of a dowser. The rod alone would not find the water, nor would the hands without the rod. But the unconscious in the dowser's body makes his muscles react minimally, and they transmit the movement to the rod, so that the conscious sees when the unconscious has discovered something.

Stories that Almost Always Work

This is not to say that it doesn't matter which stories we tell. The therapist in the mentioned example does indeed make a preselection by drawing a story from the card set and not reading out a random newspaper article. On the other hand, there are certainly stories that prove particularly effective in certain contexts and less so or not at all in others. However, there are also stories that can be used in many contexts and almost universally.

Filtration Systems

I knew an engineer who designed filtration systems. He had mainly worked for shipping companies, but also for aviation companies and NASA. "Why do you need filters on a ship?" I asked him. "For example, for cruise ships, to process the used water for reuse. The amount of water that thousands of guests consume over weeks would otherwise be too heavy to carry." "Does that mean that the water from the toilets is cleaned and goes back into the showers?" "They don't go that far—because people would find it unaesthetic. Technically, however, that would not be a problem. Such filters are used in space travel." We talked about filters for a while. Only now did I realize how diverse filters are: coffee filters that separate the powder from the tastefully and colorfully dyed water... swimming pool filters that remove insects and small parts from the bathing water... cigarette filters that let the smoke through but remove certain pollutants... water filters that can remove lime and heavy metal ions from tap water... fine dust filters that remove particles from the exhaust gases... air filters that keep the apartment clean for allergy-sensitive people. The lint screen in the washing machine is a kind of filter, as are room dehumidifiers that remove water from the air. Spring water is clean because the rock it has flowed through acts as a filter. The human body has its filters, for example the skin, which protects the inside of the body from contamination and yet has a permeability for moisture and also breathes... The stomach and intestinal wall, which lets certain substances through and others not... the kidneys, which clean the blood, the lungs, which bring oxygen into the blood, but filter out other gases and particles... then I think of the brain-blood barrier, the cell membranes... the longer I think, the more filters I find and marvel at how different their functions are. Perhaps the soul also has its filters... a filter for stressful emotions perhaps, an overload filter... one against irrelevant information... and one against things one does not want to know... a filter against boredom... Perhaps one can ask the brain to install a few additional filters, where it is needed? Or to clean the existing filters? Such filtration systems certainly also want to be cleaned from time to time... Dear brain, can you please do that? Is that possible? Yes? Thank you very much...!

Images like these can be applied in a vast spectrum of possible situations, because the client can involuntarily adapt the meanings associated with them for almost any conceivable problem. Similarly, one can talk about "valves" (Hammel 2006, p. 53, 2012, p. 49) or about the mixing console of a sound engineer (Hammel 2022, p. 217).

Stories as Greetings to the Unconscious
To instill confidence in clients that their inner selves learn involuntarily and respond to our suggestions, even if they consciously do not understand how it does so, we can also illustrate the therapeutic models we work with in a pictorial way.

The Small and the Large Self

We have a small self and a large self. The small self is what we sometimes call "consciousness" and what we usually mean when we say "I" or when we talk about what we want.

The large self is what we mean when we say "my body", "my psyche", my "unconscious", "my brain" or otherwise talk about ourselves in the third person (he, she, it) and when we talk about what happens to us, even though no one else but ourselves has done it to us.

The large self can achieve many things that the small self desires: freedom from physical symptoms, from emotional rigidity, from mental blocks and overly intense emotions.

Stories help to find words to instruct the unconscious, the body or—as we sometimes also say—the brain to work in such a way that our conscious self-experience finds peace.

Dear Brain

Sometimes it seems as if we don't know how to instruct our brain to do what we actually need. When we finally find words to ask: "Dear brain, could you do this or that for me?", it's as if the brain replies: "Sure, I can do that, no one has asked me yet!" (See also Hammel 2009, 165, 2017, 11 ff.)

Again and again, we experience inner conflicts between conscious, voluntary experience and the seemingly chaotic impulses of the unconscious, such as stress experience, affect-driven and instinctual action, traumatic dissociation, psychosomatically based diseases, etc. To illustrate how stories contribute to conflict resolution here, we can also use the metaphor of a bridge or communication in a common language.

Stories as a Bridge

The language of stories is a bridge where our goal-oriented conscious orientation and our diverse unconscious endeavors can meet, a language that both can relate to. The conscious and the unconscious can communicate in this language, just as I as a German can converse with an American or Brit in English. The other is clearly at an advantage because he speaks his mother tongue, and I probably do not grasp the nuances of what he expresses, but at least we can agree.

References

Hammel S (2006) Der Grashalm in der Wüste. Metaphern und Geschichten in Beratung, Therapie und Seelsorge. impress, Mainz

Hammel S (2009) Handbuch des therapeutischen Erzählens. Geschichten und Metaphern in Psychotherapie, Kinder- und Familientherapie, Heilkunde, Coaching und Supervision. Klett-Cotta, Stuttgart

Hammel S (2012) The blade of grass in the Desert. Storytelling: Forgotten medicine for healing the soul. A story of 100 stories for counselling and therapy. impress, Mainz

Hammel S (2017) Grüßen Sie Ihre Seele. Therapeutische Interventionen in drei Sätzen. Klett-Cotta, Stuttgart

Hammel S (2018) Handbook of Therapeutic Storytelling. Stories and Metaphors in Psychotherapy, Child and Family Therapy, Medical Treatment, Coaching and Supervision. Routledge, London

Hammel S (2019) Therapeutic Interventions in Three Sentences Reshaping Ericksonian Hypnotherapy by Talking to the Brain and Body, Routledge, London

Hammel S (2022) Hypnosystemische Therapie. Das Handbuch für die Praxis. Klett-Cotta, Stuttgart

Hammel S et al (2018) Wie das Krokodil zum Fliegen kam. 21 Therapiekarten Partnerschaft und Familie. Kurzgeschichten mit Farbfotos und einer Anleitung. Reinhardt, München

3

What Kind of Stories can I Tell?—A Shelf Full of Dreams

Trailer

This chapter distinguishes different forms of therapeutic stories. They can be exemplary or metaphorical and have positive, negative, or mysterious or open endings. There are dynamic stories with a sequence of actions in several steps, while static ones are more descriptive. Although the term "parable" would often be more appropriate than "metaphor", we use the term "metaphorical" as it has become established in the field of coaching and therapy.

To get an overview of various possibilities of therapeutic storytelling, we can categorize the stories—as well as our night and day dreams—into different categories (Hammel 2006, p. 159 f., 2009, p. 260 ff., 2012, p. 151 f., 2018, p. 217 ff., 2022, p. 222 ff., 2024).

Exemplary and Metaphorical Stories

One can distinguish between exemplary and metaphorical stories. Exemplary stories are those that have actually happened or could happen and realistically illustrate a fact based on a single event.

Metaphorical stories are those that represent a transfer from one experiential world to another and illustrate the situation being discussed in therapy in a symbolic way.

Then, one can distinguish between stories with a good ending, with a negative ending, and those with an open or mysterious ending.

In the context of therapy and coaching, metaphors are often spoken of where the term "parable" would be more appropriate. A metaphor in the true sense is a term that is "transferred" from one area of experience to another. ("Metaphor" means "carried across" and is itself a metaphor.)

A special case of exemplary stories (and a transition area to metaphors) are metonymic stories, in which a part or aspect of the situation is taken as representative of the whole. We speak of a metonymy when, for example, "Washington" is said for "the American government", "at the wheel" for "in the car" or "the crown" for "the royal family" or "the monarchy". Similarly, we can talk to clients about "your cells", "your brain" or "your insulin receptors" to illustrate complex facts—or also about constructs like "your psyche", "your unconscious", "the child in you", "your adult self", "the depression" and the like.

Static and Dynamic Stories

In a second dimension, a distinction can be made between static stories (enumerations and descriptions) with at most rudimentary dramaturgy, comparable to a meaningful photo or a collection of images (cf. "filter systems" in Chap. 2) and dynamic stories (narratives) with a fully developed sequence of actions similar to a film, cf. "Rescued Bumblebee" in Chap. 2).

Positive and Negative Learning Models—and Search Models

Most of the stories used in therapy are those with a good ending (positive learning models).

Examples are "Last will be First" and "Assisi" in Chap. 5.

Stories with a bad ending (negative learning models) can be used when the client evidently has resources that he does not use but could use—and when the story cannot be interpreted as a threat or insult, i.e. when there is a good basis of trust that excludes such an interpretation. It is advantageous if the story told has little immediate similarity to the client's life story and if it can be told with a humorous wink.

Presumably, one would not tell a client diagnosed with depression a story about a tree that stood in a wadi, in a river that only flows when it rains... Over many years it got its water again and again... but due to climate change the wadi finally dried up and the tree died... Rather, I would tell about the man who explained to me how to find water in the desert.

Finding Water

"As an engineer, I worked in Algeria and lived with the Bedouins for a few months," a friend explained to me. "At first, you're amazed at how the Bedouins always find water. You wonder how they do it. They explain to you that you have to search the sand in a desert valley for a certain shade of color, a kind of fine shadow that lies on it. That means there's water underneath. You look and look, but you don't see any shadow. But the Bedouins dig there and find water. Then I also learned to see the shadows. At

> some point, I then found a place with water that not even the Bedouins had recognized as such."

Negative learning models can still work, especially when the story is told with humor and a wink and provokes a defensive reaction in the client: "I'm not that stupid! I can do better!", without the client feeling insulted by the offer of an anti-identification figure. A friendly relationship between therapist and client, on which both sides can rely well, is a prerequisite.

Foxes and Hares

If I were the chief forester, I could take the position: "The forest is healthy when there is a maximum number of foxes"—and then wonder when there are no more hares. I could also say: "The forest is healthy when there are as many hares as possible"—then shoot all the foxes and wonder when the hares eat everything bare…

As the story is told here, it can be seen as a negative learning model or as a search model. If one wants to give the story a positive turn, one can add a concluding sentence with a friendlier outlook: "Perhaps it is better to have quite a few foxes and quite a few hares, rather than millions of foxes and no hares—or vice versa". (Another example of a negative learning model is the story "A Glass of Wind" in Chap. 7.)

Stories with an open or puzzling ending (search models) are less critical than those with a negative outcome. An open ending is recommended, among other things, when one might fear that telling a solution at the end offers too few transfer opportunities for the client, that it could therefore appear moralizing or instructive, or that the therapist with his solution offer would anticipate a decision of the client that only belongs to him.

Examples are "The Note in My Head" in Chap. 9 and "Ants" in Chap. 11.

References

Hammel S (2006) Der Grashalm in der Wüste. Metaphern und Geschichten in Beratung, Therapie und Seelsorge. impress, Mainz

Hammel S (2009) Handbuch des therapeutischen Erzählens. Geschichten und Metaphern in Psychotherapie, Kinder- und Familientherapie, Heilkunde, Coaching und Supervision. Klett-Cotta, Stuttgart

Hammel S (2012) The blade of grass in the Desert. Storytelling: Forgotten medicine for healing the soul. A story of 100 stories for counselling and therapy. impress, Mainz

Hammel S (2018) Handbook of Therapeutic storytelling. Stories and Metaphors in psychotherapy, child and family therapy, medical treatment, coaching and supervision. Routledge, London

Hammel S (2022) Hypnosystemische Therapie. Das Handbuch für die Praxis. Klett-Cotta, Stuttgart

Hammel S (2024) Transforming Lives with Hypnosystemic Therapy. A practical guide. Routledge, London

4

What Makes a Good Story?— Room for One's Own

Trailer

This chapter explains why stories that appear moralizing or instructive often lead to inner resistance in the listener. Therapeutic stories are perceived as helpful when they can be flexibly applied to the client's life. For this, even far-fetched metaphors and examples can be useful. Allegorical stories, on the other hand, offer only a limited range of interpretation and are often unfavorable for therapy. Especially example stories should not be too similar to the client's life story. This avoids false promises as well as resistance from clients who do not feel recognized when hearing about the successes or failures of other people.

Most people develop an inner resistance when the stories told to them appear moralizing or instructive. But when does a story actually appear instructive or moralizing?

© The Author(s), under exclusive license to Springer-Verlag
GmbH, DE, part of Springer Nature 2024
S. Hammel, *Learning Therapeutic Storytelling*,
https://doi.org/10.1007/978-3-662-69110-6_4

Room for Transfer

It seems to me that this is primarily the case when the story leaves little room for transfer in the listener. Therapeutic stories are usually perceived as helpful and pleasant when they offer many possibilities for how the story can be transferred to the client's life.

Clear solutions that are brought to another person from the outside without alternatives can be perceived by the listener as presumptuous or at least as not consistent.

It may play a role that people also, and perhaps especially in the area of their life interpretation, have a need for autonomy. Stories that offer a narrow range of interpretation sometimes come across as advice that ends up being blows.

With metaphorical stories, this is usually unproblematic, as the metaphorical speech already by definition requires a transfer from one area of experience to another. However, the difference between a metaphorical and an allegorical story should be kept in mind. Allegories are pictorial stories in which a transfer A = A', B = B', etc. is possible. They have more the character of examples, offer a small scope for interpretation, and are often unfavorable for therapeutic use.

An example of an allegorical story: A therapist could tell a man who is torn between his wife and his mistress about a bear who is undecided between a hike in the forest to snack on honey or to the river to fish for salmon. It is most likely to become a useful therapeutic story if the therapist carefully leaves open which option would be more advantageous for the bear and which choice he ultimately makes. Otherwise, the risk is quite high that the therapist consciously or unconsciously builds a poorly hidden bias for one of the options into such a story. The client may react obediently, angrily, or confusedly to such a story, but I suspect that he will not experience any lasting help or relief from it.

With example stories, it should be avoided that the chosen example is too similar to the client's biographical narrative. On the other hand, seemingly far-fetched examples regularly meet with positive resonance from the listeners.

You probably shouldn't tell a client with cancer stories about other people who also had cancer and got healthy. The risk that such a narrative is perceived as a cheap consolation is quite high, especially since the story could give the impression that the narrator hides a promise in it that he cannot know whether it will be fulfilled.

With a metaphor, it is more possible to address the hope for healing. Here there are more possibilities for interpretation, i.e., the therapist has put the restoration of health into the room without announcing it quite so clearly, and the clients can interpret the story for themselves as it suits them.

Assisi

I don't know if you've ever been to Assisi. There, where Saint Francis lived, they built a beautiful church. When you stand inside and look up, the ceiling is painted with a blue sky, with golden stars. Beautiful!

In 1997, there was a severe earthquake in Assisi. Many houses were damaged, and part of the sky above the church collapsed.

When the church was restored, they first removed the fragments and supported the ceiling so that no further damage could occur. Then they carefully rebuilt the damaged parts of the church. First came the masons and later the painters. If I understood correctly, they were able to use modern techniques and materials, so that the church stands more stable after the renovation than before. But the most important thing is that this wonderful church was restored, so that people can visit and admire it again, with its blue sky and golden stars.

Even metaphorical stories may appear far-fetched—that is, from areas that superficially have little to do with what the client reports.

The suggestions that the metaphorical story offers with regard to the client's situation are implemented by the client's unconscious surprisingly reliably. It is regularly noticeable that their body language expresses greater confidence after hearing metaphorically presented solution suggestions, that they express solution ideas shortly after hearing the metaphor that fit the story, and that they behave after the session as the solution offer of the metaphor suggests.

Clients usually do not ask: "What does this mean now?", but embark on an inner search and then find interesting references as to what relation the story could have to their life.

Working One-Step Removed
The American therapist Jeff Zeig, a student of hypnotherapy pioneer Milton Erickson, often noted about his teacher that he regularly worked "one-step removed from the concrete situation" in his therapy (Zeig 1995, p. 73 et seq., Hammel 2011, p. 144). Erickson often did this by telling his clients anecdotes about himself and other people he knew or had heard of. His indirect approach may have had to do with the fact that he believed, in antithesis to the psychoanalytic work then prevalent in America, that problems are not solved by bringing them to consciousness, but by having them solved by the unconscious with its much larger treasure trove of experience. Erickson believed that making burdens conscious actually hindered the work of the unconscious.

When working a step aside from the problem, another aspect seems to me to be even more significant. While we talk in therapy with people about their burdensome memories, they usually (unless we take suggestive measures to prevent this) enter the same physiological state they were in when the things they are talking about happened. In the context of therapy, this can mean panic, overwhelming grief, uncontrollable anger, but also physical, mental and emotional states of freezing, paralysis and numbness. Such conditions can firstly be very unpleasant and are also ill-suited to attitudes of wanting to understand (learning), creativity and flexibility, which are necessary for therapy. If we let people in therapy tell in detail what burdensome experiences they have had, we inadvertently put them in states that are detrimental to therapeutic learning.

Instead of going deep where each new memory threatens suffering and freezing, we can offer them—a step aside from everyday problem experiences—stories that offer their unconscious a different way of dealing with the memories, interpretations of fate and fears, which are associated with an inner mobility and an experience of creative ability.

Avalanche

Some time ago, I listened to a radio program about avalanches. A young skier said, "I always preferred to ski off the official slopes. Of course, I know you're not supposed to do that and that it can be dangerous. But for me, it was more appealing. Once, I was downhill with a friend when an avalanche broke loose beneath us. The avalanche then raced down the valley with us. We were lucky that we could stay on our skis. When we reached the valley, we were buried up to our chests in snow. We were able to dig ourselves out. It took us two hours. We then continued to walk. Eventually, we arrived at an inn where we were given warm clothes and warmed up with hot tea. I will continue to ski, even off the slopes."

This story can be told to someone who has been in danger and may have suffered damage, perhaps due to their own risky behavior. This could be someone whose marriage has broken up due to an affair or who has lost their job due to addictive behavior. The final sentence acts as an invitation to the client to consider whether they want to change their behavior or maintain their previous lifestyle. Precisely because the skier insists on maintaining his risky behavior (and the therapist does not comment on this), the story does not come across as moralizing.

References

Hammel S (2011) Handbuch der therapeutischen Utilisation. Vom Nutzen des Unnützen in Psychotherapie, Kinder- und Familientherapie, Heilkunde und Beratung. Klett-Cotta, Stuttgart

Zeig S (1995) Die Weisheit des Unbewussten. Hypnotherapeutische Lektionen bei Milton H. Erickson. Carl Auer, Heidelberg

5

How do I Find the Right Story at the Right Time?—Unearthing Treasures

Trailer

This chapter describes how therapeutic stories can be created based on idioms that clients use. Metaphors such as "shipwreck", "drowning in work" or "being trapped" can be transferred into a story to help the client solve his problem in a pictorial way. The therapist uses questions to support the client in developing an experience of confidence and ability to act. It is not necessary to return to the client's initial situation, but if the therapist does, the helpful experience of the client should be highlighted.

One of the best ways to find a therapeutically effective story at the right time is to use the client's language images, i.e., to pay attention to the idiomatic expressions (sayings) that he or she uses to describe his or her problem.

S. Hammel, *Learning Therapeutic Storytelling*, https://doi.org/10.1007/978-3-662-69110-6_5

The Clients' Metaphors

Metaphors that clients use to describe problems include the following:

- Having suffered a shipwreck,
- Drowning in work,
- A shrinking violet,
- A swamp,
- A web of lies,
- Walking on thin ice,
- Get burned,
- Being under the thumb,
- A poisoned work climate,
- Sitting high and dry,
- Being ruined,
- Being trapped,
- Being pissed off,
- Always swallowing everything,
- Hanging by a thread,
- Gut-wrenching,
- Starving someone out,
- Something is going wrong,
- Hard to stomach,
- It makes you want to tear your hair out,
- Being in a dead end,
- Being stuck in a hamster wheel,
- Choked up,
- Being put in front of a firing squad.

Exercise: Awakening the Metaphor Ear

Ask a practice partner to tell you about a situation that he is dissatisfied with, about which he is particularly annoyed or worried, for example.

Give your own unconscious the instruction beforehand to vividly bring to your consciousness every metaphor or pictorial speech like a photo. (If you like, also tell your counterpart that his unconscious should enrich his speech with a wealth of proverbial expressions, metaphors, and the like.)

Let your conversation partner speak for five to ten minutes and note the number of found language images by making strokes on a piece of paper while listening.

How many examples of pictorial speech can you identify per minute?

Give your unconscious the instruction to give you a signal in the same way during the therapy session whenever your clients use metaphors and the like!

Therapeutically Using Client Metaphors

Most of the idioms mentioned above can easily be transformed into a therapeutic story, simply by taking them literally and continuing the conversation on this basis.

If a respectful, trusting relationship between the therapist and the client is established, this can happen without a special introduction. If you want to be absolutely sure that the client notices that the therapist takes him and himself seriously and wants to change the level of conversation professionally based on a respectful attitude, you can use words to transition to the pictorial level like:

"You just said, you're on a sinking ship. If I take you quite literally, I see in my mind's eye…"

The therapist can continue:

"… you as a shipwrecked person, swimming in the water and looking for something that can save you."

With the interest in finding out how the story will continue if it has a good ending (which the therapist assumes implicitly or explicitly), he can ask questions—mostly likely W-questions (what, who, how, when…). Alternative questions often contain a therapeutically unfavorable option. So, we had better save ourselves questions like: "Can you still hold on or are you going to drown soon?" (Alternative questions with only favorable alternatives are welcome, though.) In between, the therapist can scatter in plausible information that increases the likelihood of receiving a positive (rescue-leading) answer from the client:

"In shipwrecks, there's always a lot of stuff floating around: cargo, pallets, equipment from the ship, lifeboats, lifebuoys, life jackets, etc. If you look around—what would be a suitable object nearby that you could hold on to?"

Pretty much anything the client can answer to this question will be useful to lead the story towards a good ending. The therapist can always ask further: "If we assume that the story will have a good ending, what happens next?" As a rule, the client will tell the therapist how the protagonist is saved in his imagination.

Interestingly, in the end, the client also sees himself saved and casts a confident look at his own future perspective. The metaphorically depicted problem situation originates from his own world of images, and the protagonist represents him. If the story is told coherently with the protagonist to its good end, the subconscious assumes that the same applies to the client, who was represented by the protagonist and his problem situation. Thus, his emotional state and overall physiological reactions are shaped according to the course of development that the protagonist's story takes.

And After the Story?

It is not necessary to return to the client's initial situation, i.e., the problem story that led him to therapy, after such a story. If the therapist speaks about the initial problem as if the story served only for relaxation and the problem still exists as before, he can destroy the effect of the story. It is more advantageous to let the story work involuntarily.

If the therapist still wants to return to the initial topic, it should happen in such a way that the helpful experience that the client brought from listening or co-narrating is treated as meaningful and effective, as primary compared to the previous experience. The therapist could ask with a curious-confident voice: "If you think about the initial situation again with these inner images, with this emotional experience, what is different now?"

In this way, the helpful experience—prioritized—is linked with the previous stressful experience, which is presented as secondary. The inner films of the problem experience (problem memories and problem expectations) are, so to speak, vaccinated with solution experience (solution physiology and solution emotional state).

Transforming Client Metaphors—Further Possibilities
Instead of developing such a story in dialogue, the therapist can present it monologically with equally good results. He could refer to a report of a refugee who was rescued as a shipwrecked person from the Mediterranean, or to real or fictional stories of other shipwrecked people. How did they survive? If the therapist tells this story to a good end, the effect is usually the same.

At the beginning of such an intervention, the therapist looks for a moment at what he sees in his mind's eye when he takes the image spoken of by the idiom quite literally and looks at it very vividly. If the problem image is a drowning person in the sea, he can imagine a solution image, such as an island, and in his imagination follow spatially how the client moves from the problem zone to the solution zone. If the problem zone is a desert because the client has said, "I'm drying up here," the solution zone is probably an oasis. If he feels "like in prison," the solution zone is probably the world outside the prison walls, etc. The therapist's approach is the same, only that the landscape elements are different and therefore different challenges to overcome until the protagonist (and with him the client) has arrived at a safe place.

With some idioms, it is more advantageous to imagine a timeline rather than a spatial axis. This is the case, for example, when the client himself is the problem zone, when he says, for example, "I feel like throwing up." The therapist can—perhaps again after the hint: "If you allow me to actually imagine this vividly, I see…"—point out that "throwing up" has a detoxifying function and can sometimes be experienced as liberating. He can inquire how the client deals with it when he actually feels nauseous: Does he postpone the moment of vomiting, does he want to get it over with quickly, or does he try to avoid vomiting altogether? Whether the two conduct this conversation very seriously or slightly amused, in any case a defamiliarization effect sets in: The initial topic is seen from a new perspective, and with the change of perspective, the emotional state associated with the initial topic usually improves as well.

If the client thinks he is "ruined," we can look at the image of a ruin being rebuilt in our mind's eye. Since buildings do not usually move, we also take a timeline here instead of a spatial axis. The journey leads from the problem time (ruin) to the solution time (intact building). If the client reports that he is "mired out here in the country," we can talk about buildings or agricultural areas that are "in danger of being mired", how the marsh is drained with ditches and canals and then a solid road is built into civilization. In this example, both approaches are combined: On a timeline, the village is rescued from the impending miring, on a spatial axis, a drivable road is built into civilization. The story "Assisi" in Chap. 5 shows how this narrative strategy can be applied in a monological variant.

Rule Logic

So far, we have proceeded in such a way that we take the metaphor presented by the client literally and develop it into a narrative with an action—under the assumption that the story has a happy ending. The protagonist finds the way to a better life, according to the rules that usually lead to a good outcome in the respective problem situation. Or damaged landscapes, buildings, objects are put in order, according to the rules of how this usually succeeds when it succeeds. I call this approach rule logic (cf. Hammel 2006, p. 164 f., 2009, p. 252 ff., 2012, p. 155 ff., 2022, 243 f.).

Exception Logic

Instead of rule logic, exception logic can also be used. The therapist could, for example, tell that there are several reports in maritime history of a shipwrecked person being rescued by dolphins. The fact that such a rescue is extremely unlikely usually does not bother the clients, as long as such an anecdote is presented by the therapist in a relaxed and confident manner.

If we take the metaphor "like in prison," the therapist might ask his client using the rule logic how long he still has to "serve" and when he might be released early for good behavior.

In the sense of exception logic, he can tell about a prisoner who achieved his release through legal means or who managed to escape.

Instead of telling about the restoration of a village that was destroyed by an earthquake, it can be reported how a village was rebuilt in its original form in a special case at another, safer location.

If the therapist wants to be absolutely sure that no discussion about the probability of such an event arises, which questions the intervention, he can make one or two detours after the story that temporarily distract the client's attention: He can wonder what motivates the dolphins to this behavior, note that we will probably never know, and consider what a sailor might feel after such a rescue. With the prison metaphor or the story of the relocated village, he can report on an actual case and make it plausible that the story actually happened that way. ("I saw the hole in the prison wall from the outside before they bricked it up again.")

Exercise: Transforming Problem into Solution Metaphors—Rule and Exception Logic

Meet with an exercise partner. (Feel free to greet your inner self at the beginning of the exercise, it should please provide you with a remarkably large number of proverbial expressions and other linguistic images, consciously and unconsciously, while you speak.) One of you describes (as a client) his or her annoyance about a specific interpersonal situation. The other takes these metaphorical images literally and never leaves this figurative level. He describes what he sees in his mind's eye: A protagonist in a landscape (such as a desert, a sea, or a ruin) that metaphorically represents the problem. Then he describes how the client moves from the problem zone of this landscape to a solution zone with reversed properties (such as an oasis or an island) or how the client transforms the landscape into a solution landscape (for example, by rebuilding the ruined building). For this, he either resorts to rule logic, i.e., he describes how it usually happens when this type of problem is resolved, or to exception logic, i.e., he describes how it happened exceptionally once that such a problem was resolved.

Cartoon Logic

Another possibility is the use of cartoon logic for storytelling. The therapist can, for example, communicate: "You feel 'like in prison'. If you look around, there are no iron bars, no bunk, and no high, small windows. But that's not what you meant. I just want to express: Strictly speaking, it's not you in a prison, but the prison is, so to speak, inside you, as a cartoon that your brain (or an inner director) shows you in a head cinema." With this, the therapist has done four things:

- He has noted that it is not the client, as it might have seemed, who is in the prison building, but the building is a thing within him. By swapping outside and inside, he has swapped suffering and shaping. The outside shapes the inside, the inside suffers the outside. Thus, the client has subtly moved from a position of suffering to one of shaping. To the extent that we experience an event as shaping, it can no longer traumatize us.
- He has identified the prison metaphor as an inner film. So it is distinguished from the directly experienced reality, just as a map differs from the landscape and a passport photo from the person depicted.
- By speaking of a cartoon, he has implicitly established that any change can be made to the images and the course of the film.
- He has introduced a director. This implies that an alter ego of the client has constructed the prison and can transform it into other images.

Even if not all of these implications are introduced, the cartoon technique can be used. The therapist could say: "Imagine that the prison you see before your inner eye is an image in an architect's program. You are the architect and can decide: How strong should the walls be, how large the doors, how thick and of what material the bars? How would you like to design the building so that it pleases you better?"

It is important to introduce the approach in such a way that it seems relevant and plausible to the clients to consider the metaphor as a cartoon that can be reshaped, so that the clients engage in this approach and follow it internally. Then it regularly turns out that the clients transfer the experience of the solution from the transformed problem metaphor to the experience of the solution of their initial topic. Regularly, they can then face those situations with remarkable calm, serenity, and creativity, which previously represented a great burden for them.

This approach has special advantages when clients use metaphors that are particularly destructive ("firing squad") or that have an absurd component ("gut-wrenching"). Both groups of metaphors are difficult to work with using rule logic, and the absurd metaphors are also a challenge with exception logic.

With cartoon logic, on the other hand, any kind of transformation from problem to solution situations can be designed, even if this would not be possible in reality. A castaway can pull the plug on the sea, so that the water runs out, like from a bathtub, a prisoner can escape through the keyhole, and a person dying of thirst in the desert can turn sand into water.

Exercise: Transforming Problem into Solution Metaphors—Cartoon Logic

One partner (client) describes his suffering in a situation (personal issue or role play) with proverbial expressions that denote problems. The therapist picks up on these metaphors and concretizes them by asking questions, with the aim of finding directions for solutions—or by casually pointing out inherent solutions in the image.

- How big is your golden cage? What shape does it have?
- What does the door look like? The lock?
- Is the gold real?
- You know, gold is a soft material…
- How thick or thin are the bars?
- How thick is the silk thread?
- Who and what is hanging on it?
- Do you know that silk is the strongest natural fiber in the world?
- What thickness would be necessary for greater security?
- Which knot technique?

Convey to the client in essence:

"The good thing is that it's not you in the cage (I don't see one at least), but the cage is in you. It was created in the film studio of your mind, so it can also be changed from there.

How would you like to change your cage so that it suits you better…?"

References

Hammel S (2006) Der Grashalm in der Wüste. Metaphern und Geschichten in Beratung, Therapie und Seelsorge. impress, Mainz

Hammel S (2009) Handbuch des therapeutischen Erzählens. Geschichten und Metaphern in Psychotherapie, Kinder- und Familientherapie, Heilkunde, Coaching und Supervision. Klett-Cotta, Stuttgart

Hammel S (2012) The blade of grass in the Desert. Storytelling: Forgotten medicine for healing the soul. A story of 100 stories for counselling and therapy. impress, Mainz

Hammel S (2018) Handbook of Therapeutic Storytelling. Stories and Metaphors in Psychotherapy, Child and Family Therapy, Medical Treatment, Coaching and Supervision. Routledge, London

Hammel S (2022) Hypnosystemische Therapie. Das Handbuch für die Praxis. Klett-Cotta, Stuttgart

Hammel S (2024) Transforming lives with hypnosystemic therapy. A practical guide. Routledge, London

6

How do I Structure a Therapeutic Story?—Building Stairs

Trailer

For therapeutic stories, a narrative structure in six stages is universally applicable: The (1.) protagonist is introduced, followed by (2.) his problem, (3.) his attempts at a solution, (4.) his failure, (5.) a helpful new resource, and (6.) his success. Stages 3 and 4 can be omitted, but this results in a loss of tension and the appreciation of the severity of the challenge. A story with a negative or open ending can end after stage 4 or 5.

Each model unfolds positive basic experiences as a metaphor, distributes an ambivalence to two people who transition from competition to cooperation, or traces the biographical developments of real people.

As a starting point for further experiments with therapeutic storytelling, I would like to suggest a narrative structure that is universally applicable. It works pretty much

© The Author(s), under exclusive license to Springer-Verlag GmbH, DE, part of Springer Nature 2024
S. Hammel, *Learning Therapeutic Storytelling*,
https://doi.org/10.1007/978-3-662-69110-6_6

everywhere—in fairy tales, fables, anecdotes, for telling your own experiences or for describing the experiences of other people you know or have heard about in the media.

A Good Story in six Steps

For a story with a good ending, this structure looks like this:

1. Introduce the *protagonist*!
2. Name *his problem*!
3. Describe his *attempts at a solution*!
4. Describe his *failure*!
5. Report how he discovers a new *information* or resource!
6. Tell how he experiences the desired *success* (celebration, homecoming)!

Exercise: Story-building Kit

Learn the italicized terms in their order by heart, then you have a compact kit for any story you want to tell or write.

A story with a negative ending can end after 4, one with an open ending after 5. In principle, stages 3 and 4 can also be omitted. However, this results in a loss of appreciation for the challenge the protagonist faces and the creation of tension that promotes the listener's interest. However, time is gained for other therapeutic interventions and—with skillful storytelling—a density and intensity of the description, which often makes the experience of a good punchline (surprise effect in jokes and aphorisms).

Idiomatic Stories

**Exercise: Transforming Idioms into Stories I
(Development of the Protagonist)**

Create a story from an idiom using the 6-step model.

First, pay attention to which proverbial idioms your client uses to describe their problem (and not the resource or solution).

If it is a realistically possible situation, like "being in a big mess", "spilling the milk" or "starving", vividly imagine (1) a protagonist who has this (2) problem. What does he look like? In what landscape is he and how is the problem noticeable?

What are his (3) attempts at a solution and why do they (4) fail?

Where does then (5) a new impulse, an idea, a helper or another resource that brings salvation come from? What does the (6) success look like?

Take 15 minutes to write down the story (1–2 sentences per stage)!

While the previous exercise focused on the suffering and liberation of the protagonist, we now focus on his movement in the landscape or transform the landscape in which he is located, with a similar result:

**Exercise: Transforming Idioms into Stories II
(Movement in the Landscape)**

Take the landscape idiomatically addressed by the client as an opportunity or imagine your own inner landscape photo of his problem. Then create an inner film from your inner images:

What does the problem landscape look like? Does the client see himself as…

- a "scapegoat" or "dried up", his landscape is probably a **desert**.
- a "castaway" or "drowning", his landscape is probably an **ocean**.
- "in a golden cage", "imprisoned" or "judged", his landscape is probably a **prison**.

What does the solution landscape look like accordingly? What is the opposite?

- **Oasis**
- **Island, mainland**
- **Freedom outside**

What does the path from the problem landscape to the solution landscape look like? Follow the 6 steps!

The following exercise is structured analogously to the previous one, but here it is not the protagonist moving in the landscape, but the landscape changing over time.

Exercise: Transforming Idioms into Stories III (Development of the Landscape)

Again, take the landscape idiomatically addressed by the client as an opportunity or imagine your own inner landscape photo of his problem. Then create an inner film from your inner images:

What does the problem landscape look like? Does the client see himself as…

- "ruined", "shaken", one with "many construction sites" or "destroyed", his landscape could be damaged by an **earthquake**.
- "besieged", "surrounded" or "starved", his landscape could be a city **encircled by enemies**.
- one who "could puke" or "is scared", his landscape could be a **toilet**.

Choose a solution image that is to be set after the problem image! This could be:

- the village restored later
- the city freed from enemies
- the detoxified body

What does the development from the problem landscape to the solution landscape look like? Follow the 6 steps!

In addition to the possibility of talking about metaphorical landscapes, there is also the option of drawing them alongside the conversation. Therapeutic change can be achieved by the therapist and the client jointly developing maps on which aspects of the previous problem experience and the desired solution experience are recorded.

Map Stories

Exercise: Developing Island Maps

As a therapist, consider with your client what an island would look like that symbolically represents her life situation. Would there be, for example, a volcano of anger, a swamp of lies, a lake of tears, a harbor of longing, a lighthouse of hope, etc.? Draw the outlines of an island on the flipchart. First collect 10–20 terms for such places in a list and then ask your client to draw in the respective landscape elements and names or tell you where to draw them in.

Ask where the client has recently spent a lot of time and where she would like to be more often and draw in the previous and the future desired location.

Are there neighboring islands or a mainland and should a reference to it be drawn in at the edge of the map? Should a bridge, a telephone, flight or ferry connection be established there? Consider what changes can improve life on the island (and possibly in contact with other islands or the mainland). Are roads, telephone lines, mobile phone masts, port facilities needed? Is a helicopter landing pad, a town hall or a sports facility needed? Draw the desired elements into the map.

If necessary, talk about previously experienced stresses as storms or earthquakes, which have caused damage that should now be repaired. Discuss what cleanup and renovation tasks are necessary and how the tasks should be distributed among the real or fictional cleanup workers so that the work is successful. (See Hammel 2022, 236 ff., 2024)

Stories about Fundamental Human Experiences

A simple way to structure therapeutic stories is to identify positive fundamental human experiences that can be useful to the client in their situation and to tell the client where this concept is meaningful in a completely different context.

Exercise: Using Metaphors of Fundamental Human Experiences

Ask yourself or the client during the anamnesis conversation or during the goal and assignment clarification, which characteristic or ability your client would like to have or which would be useful to him to achieve his goal. What is a simple word for the fundamental experience that he may need more than before?

Learning? Searching? Waiting? Maturing? Defending oneself? Saving oneself in time?

Find such a central term for what your counterpart needs in silence. Look in which area of nature, technology, professional practice, and social life this term still plays a central role. Tell your counterpart everything that can be said about it in this other area. So:

- If it's about learning, tell about elementary school, driving school, or dance school.
- If it's about searching, tell about Easter eggs, hide and seek, or partner search.
- If it's about waiting, tell about Santa Claus or experiences in the waiting room.
- If it's about maturing, tell about the ripening of fruits or vegetables, etc.

Then discuss the effect of the procedure on the client's experience.

Biographical Stories

Another possibility is to tell stories about real people who have overcome a crisis and subsequently experienced rescue or success. Such a story should, as mentioned, not be too similar to the client's life story and should not appear trivial or overly successful in a way that the client might feel not taken seriously in his current stress.

Exercise: Telling Biography Excerpts as Solutions

Tell a snippet from an artist, explorer, or inventor biography you know from a critical point to success or the story of a survivor from acute danger to rescue. Consider: What resource led to success or rescue? Anecdotes may have a legendary character. So feel free to reduce the story to a few central aspects and embellish it imaginatively from these core points!

In child and adolescent therapy, there is the possibility to inquire about the child's career dream or which media stars it admires. If the child wants to become a footballer, a story about an aspiring football professional can be told, if it wants to become a vet, a story about a young veterinarian.

If the child's challenge is to come to class regularly and on time, not to react physically violently to verbal provocations, or not to steal anymore, this topic is linked to a representative of the mentioned profession. When telling the story, any devaluation of the protagonist and also a broad (possibly enjoyable) spread of failure is avoided to avoid unnecessary moralization of the topic. Instead of the previously presented six-step scheme, a four-step one can be chosen:

1. The aspiring professional shows the behavior considered problematic.
2. He experiences how failure results from it in his profession and is frustrated.
3. An experienced representative of his profession shows him how to master the situation.
4. He tries out this approach and is successful with it.

As a 5th step, it can be told how the same person later as a trainer helps other job starters with the initially identified problem to succeed.

Exercise: The Path to Full Mastery

Think of a child in your therapeutic practice who has a social problem to cope with!

Consider what hobbies and interests it has and which profession is particularly associated with it.

Choose a representative of this profession and tell how this person has overcome a problem that is similar or identical to that of the child.

The elaboration of such a story can follow the scheme described above in a few sentences or be designed more complexly, as the following example shows.

The Fastest and Strongest Submarine in the World

A clever inventor wanted to build the strongest and fastest submarine in the world. To make it really fast, he omitted any component that he didn't absolutely need. When he finished building it, he immediately tested it. On its first voyage, it hit a rock. Severely damaged, his submarine had to resurface. It took a while for him to repair it. "What do you think I did wrong?" he asked a friend who was also an inventor. "Maybe you should install windows and headlights so you can see where you're going," the friend said. So the inventor installed windows and headlights in his submarine. On the second dive, he hit a ship. The steering was damaged and he had to resurface urgently. "What do you think was the mistake?" he asked his friend. "I think you should install a brake," he said. So the inventor installed a brake in his submarine. On the third dive, he hit a ship with his submarine again. This time he had to surface his boat with engine damage. "What do you think was the mistake now?" he asked his friend. "I think you should install a radar system or sonar system," he replied. So the inventor installed a radar and a sonar system in his submarine. On the fourth dive, it didn't hit anything anymore. However, the inventor got lost underwater and didn't know where he was when he surfaced. "What do you think was the mistake?" he asked his friend. "I think you should install a navigation system," was the answer. So the inventor installed a navigation system in his submarine. The fifth time, he was able to travel very far and didn't get lost anymore. However, the people above water didn't know where he was or if he was still alive. After a while, they lost interest in his excursion and left. "What do you think was the mistake?" he asked his friend again after surfacing. "I think you should install a radio system, some kind of underwater mobile phone, so you can stay in contact with the people above water while you're submerged." So the inventor installed a radio system in his submarine. On the sixth dive, nothing broke anymore, he no longer got lost underwater, he stayed in radio contact with the people above water. By now his submarine was no longer the fastest in the world, but still very fast—above all, it no longer broke, he always knew where he was, could talk to the people above water at any time and therefore had a lot of fun on his underwater trips. (See Hammel 2009, p. 162 ff.)

This story can be used, among other things, with children with social abnormalities, such as in the context of an ADHD diagnosis. It contains suggestions for improving the perception of the environment, social behavior, motor control, self-assessment, and communication. It is implied that the child does not need to stop dreaming, being in motion, loving power and speed, and that it does not need to change anything about its personality. Its unconscious should achieve a reduction of conflicts with the environment with as few targeted adjustments of its behavior and experience as possible. Otherwise, it can maintain its somewhat unusual attention style (the "diving").

In therapy, the story will not be told in full length, but will be adapted to fit as closely as possible to the challenges of the individual child.

A simple story can also be created by focusing on when the client has mastered a crisis in a completely different previous situation, experienced a time of success, or achieved a very special success.

The client is then addressed to this experience and asked to tell about it. The therapist can ask him how he achieved the surprisingly good result or tell about others who have achieved such successes and point out that the client himself is an example of such experiences.

This narrative structure is also suitable for seemingly trivial life experiences such as learning to read, learning to drive a car, teaching a child to walk, climbing trees, recovering from an infection, etc.

Exercise: The Times of Success

When the client describes a problem that has a good chance of being solved, think about where in the past he has definitely learned something, overcome something, or successfully coped with something.

You can refer to individual experiences that the client has told you about, to learning steps that he has obviously mastered (learning to speak, learning to walk, depending on how he came to the session, bus or car driving), to professional or private successes (e.g. in sports or in an artistic activity).

Exchange ideas in a jointly developed story about how the client and other people (in a very modest presentation of your own experiences possibly also yourself) have managed to go through this development.

Discuss with the client how his mood in relation to the initial problem changes in the process.

Principle Stories

What principles do you use to shape your counseling? Would these principles also be useful for your clients in their respective situations?

Perhaps you act according to the principle: Self-protection comes first, then care for others! Then you could tell a client the following story:

Safety Regulation

"Good morning. On behalf of the flight captain and the crew, we warmly welcome you on board Flight 714 from Frankfurt to Madrid..." The stewardess's voice sounded friendly and routine. As she wished, I put my seat upright and fastened my seatbelt. Then I looked out the window, where the runway seemed to slowly move backward. I heard the friendly voice say, "Should there be a loss of cabin pressure during the flight, an oxygen mask will automatically drop from the panel above your seat. With the help of the attached rubber band, you can tighten the mask on your head. Press the mask firmly against your face and breathe deeply and calmly. Travelers with small children should put on their own mask *first* and take care of their child's safety *afterwards*..." I looked next to me, where my two-year-old was snuggled in her blanket. I wondered: Would I follow this regulation? (Hammel 2006, p. 44, 2012, p. 40)

You could design your work according to a second principle: I do not focus on the problem, but on the exceptions to the problem. Then I consider which contexts condition the emergence of these exceptions and promote the contextual conditions in which these resources thrive. Then I focus on how the newly emerged resources (i.e., the initial exceptions to the problem) can be secured and extended into other areas. Then you could tell your clients the following story:

The Blade of Grass in the Desert

A man was crossing a desert. All around him there was only sand, stones and rocks, the bright blue sky and above him the scorching hot sun. Halfway through his journey, he wanted to rest and looked for a suitable place. A little off the path, he found an overhanging rock that could provide him with shade for his rest. The man went there. When he arrived, he saw something unusual: In the shadow of this rock, a blade of grass was actually growing. "Well, where did you come from?" the man asked, and then he laughed at himself: "In my loneliness, I'm already talking to the grass. It would be better if I investigated where the blade of grass comes from." He scraped the plant out of the sand and carefully put it aside. Then he dug deeper and deeper. Even though he did not hit a gushing spring, the earth here was indeed somewhat moist. When the man continued on his way, he did not forget to put the blade of grass back on the moist earth. With a few stones, he built a small wall in front of it to protect the plant from drying out due to the hot desert wind. Then he continued his journey. On his way back, he passed the spot again. Of course, he checked whether his plant was still alive. He was very pleased: The blade of grass had become a proper little grass bush. The man dug a little deeper into the earth and reached even moister soil. With a cloth, two stakes, and a few ropes that he had taken for the return journey, he improved the wind protection for his plant. Many years later, a friend of this man had to cross the same desert. He asked the friend: "Could you check what happened to my plant—if it's still there?" The friend promised him. When he returned from the trip, he reported: "Your grass bush has become a small piece of meadow. Other travelers have discovered the spot. They have enlarged the wall and set up more stakes with cloths there. Someone has dug a well there and covered it with a piece of leather. Next to the well, a beautiful fig tree is growing. A cricket was chirping in its leaves". (Hammel 2006, pp. 77 f., cf. Hammel 2012, p. 73)

Ambivalence Stories

Another way to work with stories is to distribute an ambivalence in which the client finds himself to two or more people (Hammel 2009, pp. 309 ff.). There are basically several possibilities.

Option 1: The people can represent the contextual conditions for the success or failure of a project, with one person standing for success and one or more for failure.

The Scent of Bread

"Woman," said the baker, "I am getting older and my strength is fading. I have baked bread for this village all my life. Yes, people have come from afar to buy my rolls. When the day comes that I have to put down the dough bowl, who will continue the business?" The two had no children. "Go," said the woman, "find a young man who can assist you, and whom you can teach everything about your craft. When you are old and can no longer work, he should continue the shop and you should be proud of him as if he were a son." So the baker spread the word in the surrounding villages that he was looking for someone who liked to bake bread and wanted to learn this craft from him. In the following days, four young men presented themselves to him, and he had the agony of choice. And since the decision was difficult for him, he went to his wife and asked her. She said, "Bring them all back. I will tell you which one to choose." Said and done. The baker had the four men come again. The first man introduced himself, and she asked him, "Why do you want to become a baker?" "I like to get up early and go to bed early. And a baker learns all the news in the village and the surrounding area early on." The second came, and she asked him, "Why do you want to become a baker?" "My parents have passed away, and I have a wife and children to support."

The third came, and she asked him, "Why do you want to become a baker?" "I consider it an honor to bake the bread that God has given us." The fourth came, and she asked him nothing. "We'll take him," she said to her husband.

"And why him?" "When he came in, he deeply inhaled the scent of the bread." (Hammel 2006, p. 28; cf. Hammel 2012, p. 26)

Option 2: The individuals can represent two different strategies for realizing needs, living values, overcoming crises, or achieving successes. The following story focuses on two people whose attitudes to life exemplify possible attitudes that a client can adopt.

Two Paths to Happiness

"What can I do to be happy someday? Is there a path to happiness, and if so, how can I find it?" I asked myself. It was a time when I was very unhappy. So I wondered who among my friends and acquaintances was the happiest person. If I could find out how he did it, it might help me become a happier person myself. Of course, happiness cannot be proven, but who did I consider the happiest? The happiest person seemed to me to be a man named Hugo—although at first glance he didn't seem to have much reason to be happy. His mother had died in a car accident when he was fourteen, his father had been murdered a few years later on a holiday trip. He had dropped out of an electrician's apprenticeship and a study program, then worked in the beverage trade and a delivery service until he was retired early due to an accident. Hugo loved to read novels and listen to audiobooks, to cook for his wife, to program computer programs, and to repair broken things. He learned Spanish and French and dealt with scientific and philosophical questions.

Of course, Hugo could have been unhappy. He could have pondered why his parents had died early, why he had not completed any training, why his cat had been run over, why he himself had suffered a serious accident, had to retire early, and much more. Hugo did none of that. Hugo was content—with himself, with his life, with the world as it was. Being content with the way things are—that's one path to happiness. Hugo was the person in my environment who mastered the art of contentment best.

The person I considered the second happiest was Annegret. She always had a goal, and if she didn't have one, she looked for one that she believed she could achieve. She pursued her goal with all her energy. When she achieved it, she celebrated her success, took a little break, set the next goal, and pursued it until she achieved it and could celebrate her success. If something got in her way on the path to her goal, she didn't blame herself or others. She only asked what she could contribute to make it succeed better next time. And if the achievement of her goal was completely thwarted by adverse circumstances, she didn't blame herself either, but looked around again and sought a new, achievable goal.

These are the paths to happiness I have found. It is possible that the happiest people in the world are those who walk on both paths.

There are a lot of people who do it a bit like Annegret, but then again differently, and I don't count them among the happy people. They look for a goal, pursue it, achieve it, and look for the next goal. They just always forget one thing....

Option 3: The individuals can represent two impulses for action that the client experiences and that have so far hindered or blocked each other.

Try this option yourself! Test several variants...

Exercise: Transformation of an Ambivalence Conflict as a Cartoon—the Client as Director

The client describes an ambivalence. The therapist invites the client to imagine the options facing each other as cartoon characters. Who are they? What do they look like?

How do they behave individually or in relation to each other? The therapist invites to change the scene…

The therapist now invites the client to freely modify the image using cartoon techniques, so that a solution becomes possible in the new image, e.g.

- the exterior or
- the behavior of the characters,
- their size or
- position to each other.

Discuss what has changed for the client after the exercise!

Ambivalence conflicts experienced internally by clients can also be resolved by bringing the two sides of the ambivalence into conversation and winning them over to pursue a common strategy. It is recommended that the client leaves it to the ambivalent sides to see which strategies they find. In this way, the client's unconscious finds an implementation strategy that his conscious would often not be capable of.

Exercise: Transformation of an Ambivalence Conflict as Mediation—The Client as Appreciative Boss of His Options

The client describes an ambivalence. The therapist invites the client to imagine the options facing each other as differently appearing clones of himself (as externalized "parts") or cartoon characters.

- The therapist points out that both want something good, perhaps even the same thing, and only have different strategies for implementing this value.
- Unfortunately, they block each other—as a team they could achieve more.

- He asks if they understand this and if they will commit as a team for the client.
- He asks the client to describe how they talk to each other or adjust their behavior to each other and to the client's needs.

Of course, ambivalences can also be represented as a story with a dramaturgy from problem to solution. Such a story can be designed according to the 6-step model, with two protagonists on the way to a solution instead of one acting person. The decisive impulse for problem solving can then come from a third person or from a common discovery of the protagonists.

Exercise: Transformation of an Ambivalence Conflict as Drama—The Client as Witness to the Solution of an External Conflict

The therapist tells a story according to the 6-step model, but this time with two protagonists instead of one, onto whom the conflict is distributed. The positions of the two are equally appreciated, so they are not presented according to a right-wrong scheme. Both protagonists are "right" in their value system, and yet their behavior seems to exclude each other. An unexpected discovery or an advisor entering the scene finally allows a solution.

The therapist or the client names from the conversation about the conflicting inner impulses...

- **two protagonists**: Into what time and environment do they fit?
- **a problem**: For which values or needs do the protagonists stand? With what practical implementation strategies do they seek to meet these? What conflict do they have and how do they carry it out?
- **various attempts at solution**: What solutions have they tried individually or together? Which ones have they not even tried?
- **the failure**: How does the failure show and how do the two react to it?

- **a decisive new impulse**: What kind of helper figure can be helpful here? What does she say or do? How does movement now come into the matter?
- **A solution**: How do the protagonists react when it becomes clear that this works? How does their life change as a result? How do they celebrate?

Alienation Stories

Another way to create metaphorical stories that can help solve problems is to reframe the life situation in which a person feels burdened, and to view one's own life from a helpfully different perspective. The following exercises can be used for a self-experiment, but are also explicitly intended to be given to clients as "homework". I use them primarily in child and adolescent therapy, but they are also suitable for adults.

For example, we can perceive life as a computer game. Those who are not familiar with the current games or want to simplify the method (and thus save time-consuming excursions) can talk about the simple computer games from earlier times like Pac-Man, Tetris or Space Invaders (see "Pac-Man" in Hammel et al. 2018, 40 f. and "Playing Tetris" in Hammel et al. 2021, 43 f.). Similarly, we can invite clients to imagine their life as a movie…

Exercise: Life as a Movie

Do you sometimes feel annoyed at your workplace? Imagine your job is the location for a new movie and everyone is busy rehearsing their role. Some have already mastered their role very well, while others still need a lot of practice. Only now do you realize why some people behave so strangely: It's not really their way, but just the role they are preparing for. Look around and you might recognize the producer, the director, and the makeup artist and be able to better understand their behavior, which you sometimes wondered about.

A stressful life situation can also be reframed by changing the job description so that something enjoyable, previously considered completely incidental, is declared the main thing, while the unpleasant aspects, which were previously considered the really important thing, are only treated as a peripheral aspect of the actual work.

Exercise: Life as a Psychological Study

Imagine your work task is actually part of a psychological study. In it, you are to show that people who are smiled at by you at work are less prone to unfriendly behavior than people who are treated neutrally (control group). Alternatively, you could be tasked with chatting with friendly people and delighting in the beauty of the room decoration and some people, while you are busy with various activities that others might mistakenly think are the actual purpose of your work. It could also be your task to pretend intensively that your work is intelligent or important and even fun. (See www.stefanhammel.de/blog/2007/11/06/329)

Another possibility is to transform the stressful life situation mentally into a sporting challenge. For this, we base it on a sport or another activity with a competitive character that the client himself practices or identifies with.

I had a boy play a football game against boredom (Hammel 2014, 94 ff.), I asked a horse-loving girl to imagine the tasks as hurdles in show jumping, a ballet enthusiast I asked if there were competitions with a jury in her field. We thought together about what a concept would have to look like where she goes through several dance performances and each time gets the maximum score from several jury members. I suggested the following to a teenager who found it difficult to concentrate on homework:

Doing Homework in the Mountains

I asked a boy who loved mountain hikes to print out a hiking map of a summit tour he had already done, a map with contour lines.

If he has to solve 10 math homework problems, he should make a cross on the path he has taken, counting down from the summit, every 100 meters in altitude, so that ten tasks correspond to a thousand meters in altitude.

After each task, he could, figuratively speaking, take a drink break: circle the corresponding cross, pause for a few minutes, look around with his inner eye and remember what it looked like at that point. After 500 or 600 meters in altitude, it would be time for a small snack break with a bit more time to look around and pause, and at the summit, after 1000 meters, for a big break with a bar of chocolate, fruit, peanuts or whatever he would have as provisions in such a case.

Another way to work with therapeutic stories is to create personified resources, some would also say: helper figures.

Exercise: Invisible Friends

Work together as a therapist and client. The client describes his suffering in a situation. As a therapist, consider what resource he needs to cope with the situation: courage, creativity, health, generosity, flexibility?

Ask or consider what this resource would look like personified. Who or what could best embody it? Or consider what the perfect helper would look like in this situation: Would it be the deceased mother, a troll, Einstein, a robot, a tree, or the conversation partner himself as a wise old man/wise old woman?

Or turn it into a dialogue:

- Start a conversation about children's invisible friends, about experiences with such helpers and books in which they appear.
- Ask the client what his optimal helpers would look like and what they would do.

- Fabricate stories together about living with this figure.
- Talk to him about how he can use his helper.
- Suggest talking to the helper, asking him questions and praising him.

References

Hammel S (2006) Der Grashalm in der Wüste. Metaphern und Geschichten in Beratung, Therapie und Seelsorge. impress, Mainz

Hammel S (2009) Handbuch des therapeutischen Erzählens. Geschichten und Metaphern in Psychotherapie, Kinder- und Familientherapie, Heilkunde, Coaching und Supervision. Klett-Cotta, Stuttgart

Hammel S (2012) The blade of grass in the desert. Storytelling: Forgotten medicine for healing the soul. A story of 100 stories for counselling and therapy. impress, Mainz

Hammel S (2014) Therapie zwischen den Zeilen. Das ungesagt Gesagte in Psychotherapie, Beratung und Heilkunde. Klett-Cotta, Stuttgart

Hammel S (2018) Handbook of therapeutic storytelling. Stories and metaphors in psychotherapy, child and family therapy, medical treatment, coaching and supervision. Routledge, London

Hammel S (2022) Hypnosystemische Therapie. Das Handbuch für die Praxis. Klett-Cotta, Stuttgart

Hammel S (2024) Transforming lives with hypnosystemic therapy. A practical guide. Routledge, London

Hammel S et al (2018) Wie der Bär zum Tanzen kam. 120 Geschichten für einen gesunden Körper. Reinhardt, München

Hammel S et al (2021) Wie der Tiger lieben lernte. 120 Geschichten zum Umgang mit psychischem Trauma. Reinhardt, München

7

Where to Connect, Where to Lead?—Stops in the Landscape of Life

Trailer

People come to therapy when they are at a low point and fear that it may stay that way or get even worse. The therapist chooses a protagonist as an identification figure who is also in a crisis. A story is then told that leads from a low point to a high point and follows the rules of the chosen narrative genre, so that no objections arise in the client. The protagonist can either be a real or fictional person, the client himself at an earlier stage of life, the therapist, a well-known person, or a possible or evidently unreal figure invented by the therapist.

Life is a series of ups and downs, and people usually come to therapy when they have reached a low point in their life curve and fear that the course of the curve may stay in this zone for a longer time or could even point further downwards.

Since the client is in a crisis, i.e., at a low point in his life, the therapist will choose a protagonist as an identification figure who is also in a crisis.

From there, the therapist will usually tell the story in such a way that it logically leads from the initial low point to a high point. How such a story can be structured was explained in Chap. 6 "Building Stairs". It is essential that this story is told in such a way that at no point does a no-impulse arise in the client, i.e., an objection in the sense of "That doesn't fit!" or "That's not possible at all!" This is usually ensured if the rules of the initially chosen narrative genre are maintained.

This means: In a fairy tale, it doesn't bother if people cast spells and animals talk, but it might if they perform centrifugal force calculations. In a report on the development of the first moon rocket, centrifugal force calculations can occur, but magic spells and talking animals are rather unlikely.

The Protagonists of a Therapeutic Story
Real or fictional persons can be protagonists:

- The client himself with a previous life experience,
- The therapist with his own experience,
- Someone the therapist knows,
- A real person known from history or the media,
- A fictional person known from movies, books, or other media,
- A person invented by the therapist, either fairy-tale-like or realistically possible.

I would like to give an example for each of these variants.

Playing the Piano

In supervision, someone asked me: "How do you learn what you do: Paying attention to facial expressions and gestures, to the voice and intonation and speech rhythm, and then still listening to what the client is saying?"

"I heard you play the piano. How do you learn that? I believe, you first learn to use the left hand and then the right and then both hands in interaction with each other. Then you learn how to use the left foot and how to coordinate its activity with the right and left hand. At one time you will take care of the dynamics, at another time of the touch and again at another time of aspects of expression, of pauses and syncopations. You will also not concentrate on acquiring the basic motor skills and learning to read music at the same time, but will direct your attention once to one and then to the other, to finally network both, the motor skills and the reading of music. At some point, you can play a piece of music and listen to a conversation that others are having in the same room at the same time."

The story serves to win the supervisee over to the view that he already applies the ability he wants to acquire in another area. He can and will learn what he needs and already has a good experiential basis for it. Instead of playing the piano, driving a car could serve as an example. In similar contexts, Milton Erickson used learning to speak (Rosen 2000, p. 54 f., 69), learning to walk (Short, Weinspach 2007, p. 18 f.) or learning to swim (Rosen 1982) as illustrative examples from the experiential world of his conversation partners.

The Last will be First

As a child, I was quite scatterbrained. One day I thought school would start with the second hour. But I had mixed up the day. School started with the first hour, and in the first two hours a math test was written. I arrived in class when the first hour was already well advanced and made a sincere effort to catch up with concentration and fast writing. Some time before the end of the second hour, the teacher looked over my shoulder and said loudly: "That's strange—Stefan was the last to arrive and is now one of the first to finish."

I use the story to win people over to the view that delays in pursuing personal or professional goals can also be used to pursue the set goals with even greater determination and possibly achieve them even better.

With Both Eyes

Many years ago, a man came to me for therapy because he was afraid of losing an eye. They had cut a tumor out of his face and told him, "We hope it stays away. If it comes back, we will have to cut out a larger area and then also amputate your eye." We worked on him being able to deal with this announcement as fearlessly and calmly as possible. Unfortunately, the tumor came back. They then cut out a larger piece and also removed the eye. He called me from the hospital to arrange a new appointment. Three weeks after the surgery, he sat in front of me with bandages on his face and said, "Don't worry about my eye. I tell all my friends: I still have both eyes: Seeing is a matter of the mind, and the mind is produced in the brain. If both eye areas in the brain are still there, then the eyes are still there for my brain. And if they are still there for my brain, i.e., my mind, they are still there for me. The eye is not a problem for me. Can we do something about the eczema?"

I tell this story to some people who have suffered a loss to illustrate: You don't need to say goodbye more than absolutely necessary. The physical encounter is no more, but the invisible relationship and thus the encounter in the mind, may remain.

> **The Goldmaker**
>
> In olden times, a man lived among us who belonged to the class of those who call themselves alchemists, he boasted that he had found a way to make gold. When the king of that land heard this, he summoned the man and asked him to share this secret. The man now vainly asserted that he knew nothing of such an art. "Then I will lock you up as a liar and deceiver," said the king, "For either you are one, because you claimed to others that you could make gold, although you cannot, or you are one, because you assert to me that you cannot, although you actually master this art. Just tell me what you need to make gold. You will get it in your dungeon. As soon as you are done, you may announce it—and if you tell us how you put it into practice, you shall be set free." The poor man now had plenty of time to try something. One day he told the jailer, "I have discovered something." "And what would that be?" asked the latter. "I have discovered the secret art by which the Chinese produce the porcelain they sell to our royal court for much gold." The jailer reported this to the king, and he summoned the prisoner. When the prisoner had reported his discovery, the king declared, "You have not invented gold, but something that is more than that. From this day on, you shall be free." With that, he released him from his dungeon, dressed him like a nobleman, and presented him with royal gifts. (Hammel 2006, p. 49, 2012, p. 45)

The story tells, with poetic license, a snippet from the biography of the alchemist Johann Friedrich Böttger (1682–1719), who claimed to be able to make gold, was held captive by King August the Strong, and during his imprisonment discovered with other scientists of his time how to make porcelain.

Anecdotes from the life of a legendary or historical person are also the stories "Scylla and Charybdis", "A Miracle in Stages" and "No Miracle" in Chap. 13.

Dementors

Do you know what Dementors are? It is said that they are spirits that settle on people and confuse them so that they no longer know where they come from and where they want to go.

  Imagine you have a following of a hundred Dementors. You can throw one at anyone who annoys you. Then they will be confused and distracted and forget what they were about to do. You don't need to use them all at once—you might want to keep a few in reserve. Who would you use your first Dementors on and what, do you imagine, will then happen?

The idea of Dementors comes from the novel Harry Potter, where it is described that they suck happiness, emotions, and life energy from other people. The Dementors presented here are milder than the original version, they only confuse the other person and thus protect the one who sends them out. It doesn't hurt if the client knows the version from the book. The imagined power to sic a terrifying spirit like a trained dog on an opponent contributes to self-confidence and thus to the ability to deal with hostilities sovereignly.

The story can not only be used for the imaginative change of threateningly experienced people, but can be applied to any fear situation.

A Jar of Wind

In China, there lived a man who had captured the wind in a preserving jar. To all visitors he said, "I've got it. It's in there." Many came and left shaking their heads. They had not felt a fresh breeze. Some asked him, "What do you want with the empty jar?" And he proudly explained, "When I need wind, I just open the jar, and whoosh, a cool breeze goes through the room. For example, when I have guests in my attic apartment in the summer: 'Uff, it's hot in here,' they groan, and I say 'Just a moment, we'll have that sorted out.' A simple gesture—and a fresh breeze sweeps through the room. Or if something has burned while cooking: With a jar of wind, all smells are quickly swept away."

Some said, "Open the jar!" But he replied, "For God's sake! Then all the wind is gone. And what should I do with the jar then?" (Hammel 2006, p. 75 f., 2012, p. 71)

The story can be told to people who unconsciously maintain old protective mechanisms when they are no longer useful, to invite their unconscious to adapt or abandon these strategies. Examples are phobic avoidance strategies, freezing reactions (depersonalization, depression) or social withdrawal. The story is an example of a negative learning model. The client is invited to protest, either aloud or silently: I'm not that stupid! It is important to tell the story on the basis of a trusting, appreciative relationship with humor and a wink. Similarly oriented is the story "Date Expired" in Hammel (2009, p. 189, cf. Hammel 2018), which is about the tendency of some people to store food in the refrigerator until it is clearly no longer edible.

References

Hammel S (2006) Der Grashalm in der Wüste. Metaphern und Geschichten in Beratung, Therapie und Seelsorge. impress, Mainz

Hammel S (2009) Handbuch des therapeutischen Erzählens. Geschichten und Metaphern in Psychotherapie, Kinder- und Familientherapie, Heilkunde, Coaching und Supervision. Klett-Cotta, Stuttgart

Hammel S (2012) The blade of grass in the Desert. Storytelling: Forgotten medicine for healing the soul. A story of 100 stories for counselling and therapy. impress, Mainz

Hammel S (2018) Handbook of therapeutic storytelling. Stories and metaphors in psychotherapy, child and family therapy, medical treatment, coaching and supervision. Routledge, London

Hammel S (2022) Hypnosystemische Therapie. Das Handbuch für die Praxis. Klett-Cotta, Stuttgart

Hammel S (2024) Transforming lives with hypnosystemic therapy. A practical guide. Routledge, London

Rosen S. (ed.) (1982). My Voice Will Go with You. Teaching Tales of Milton H. Erickson. Norton, New York

Short D, Weinspach C (2007) Hoffnung und Resilienz. Therapeutische Strategien von Milton H. Erickson. Carl Auer, Heidelberg

8

Where do I Start and How do I Continue?—The Wrong English

Trailer

Therapeutic storytelling can be done with simple anecdotes and in everyday language. It is not necessary for the story to be perfect in a literary sense, as the therapeutic effect does not depend on this. What is important is that the story fits into the context of the therapy and contributes to the processing of the client's concerns. To this end, it is useful to adapt stories to current needs by shortening, embellishing, or individually modifying them. The same story can also be meaningful in completely different contexts. When one story is finished, another can be told that expands or complements the meaning of the first.

"How do I start with therapeutic storytelling?", someone might ask. "What's stopping you from starting?", I would ask back. Put differently: What actually prevents us from telling bad stories? For starters, until they perhaps get better someday... whatever "better" might mean...

© The Author(s), under exclusive license to Springer-Verlag
Gmbh, DE, part of Springer Nature 2024
S. Hammel, *Learning Therapeutic Storytelling*,
https://doi.org/10.1007/978-3-662-69110-6_8

After all, it's not about what we tell our clients having to appear in printed form. We don't even need to solemnly present the anecdotes we tell as "stories", thus exposing them to theoretically possible criticism.

The Wrong English

A German family traveled to America. The mother was American, and the children were finally going to meet their relatives. The younger daughter had only had two years of English lessons. She made many mistakes, but she talked incessantly. She got along well with her uncles, aunts, cousins, and had a lot of fun with them. The older one had already been learning English for three years. She tried not to make any mistakes. To speak correctly, she always took a little longer to think. Often the conversation had moved on by the time she knew what she wanted to say. So, she mostly said nothing.

When the family set off for home after a few weeks, the younger daughter was happy, but the older one was crying heavily. "Are you sad because the vacation is over?", asked her mother. "That's not it," the girl replied. "I feel like I didn't get to know my relatives at all. I didn't want to make any mistakes, and then I didn't say anything at all."

Experience shows that the effect of therapeutic stories does not depend on their literary quality.

We can present our story in exactly the same tone in which we would tell friends on the phone or at dinner about what happened to us today or what we read in a magazine. What harm could come to us or the clients from this? However, the clients could certainly benefit from the story. As mentioned, they came to therapy to find help and will involuntarily search what they heard for its contribution to the processing of their concerns. The story takes on a different, deeper meaning in this context than if it were told among friends in the evening.

Perhaps I would tell the following memory to the person who asked me how to start storytelling…

Learning to Hypnotize

There were 23 participants in my hypnotherapy training group. At the beginning, we practiced how to induce a hypnotic trance in another person, later it was about therapeutic techniques. Everything I learned, I immediately tried out at home with other practice partners, changed it, varied it, and thus expanded my skills. A few courses and months later, my impression was that I was the only one in the group who had learned hypnosis in its classic form. Most participants, it seemed to me, had postponed practicing until they had learned more basics and acquired more skills. And while they were always learning new things, the old ones were constantly fading.

If we apply what we learn immediately, there is a high probability that we can consolidate and retain it. If we vary, process, transfer, and transform what we have learned in some way, there is a high probability that we can expand what we have gained.

Perhaps it would like to be processed in the brain once or twice:

- What is heard can be written down, what is written can be spoken again.
- Handwritten notes can be typed into the computer and typed notes can be handwritten.
- What is learned in German can be reproduced in English, standard language can be translated into dialect and vice versa.
- Thoughts can be spoken. What is said is heard and what is heard is thought again.

- Words can be translated into actions or into panto-mimic forms of expression and vice versa.
- What is spoken can also be whispered, shouted, or sung.

The Note in My Head

In the copy room of our university library, there was a note: "Copying is better than studying". I found that quite funny. Today, three decades later, I wonder why I still think about this sentence. I still wonder what this sentence was supposed to mean…

If things are learned and consolidated particularly well by processing them in different ways, it will also be useful to sometimes transfer stories from one form to another and from one context to another.

Long stories can be shortened to their core and short ones can be embellished further. Landscapes and objects can be exchanged and the sequence of events may also be changed.

Stories that we have used so far for mental stress can be adopted into the therapy of physical illnesses or into the processing of interpersonal conflicts. Stories that we have used in the therapy of physical stress can be adopted into couple therapy or for the processing of inner psychological conflicts, and stories that we initially told to groups can be used to regulate body functions.

After the Storytelling

The next question that seminar participants often ask is: "What do I do when the story is over? How do I continue then?" The simplest answer is: "Then you tell another story that complements and expands the first one in its mean-ing." If this story is only a thematic variation on the first, i.e., it says almost the same thing in different words, then it reinforces the message of the first story. If it goes in a different direction, it complements the message of the first story with another aspect. If it goes in roughly the opposite direction as the first, the impression is created that the two stories juxtapose different views and action options, each of which has its right and place.

Thus, the story "Learning to Hypnotize" primarily had the function of reinforcing the previous story "The Wrong English" in its meaning. At the same time, it brought a new aspect to the fore: "What is learned and immediately continued is usually retained; what is learned and not immediately continued is usually lost."

Seminar participants often ask: "What do I answer when a client asks me: 'What do you want to tell me with this story?'"

It seems to me unfavorable to dissolve the complexity of a story, which can lead people into searching, in favor of a simple answer that ends the search. So I would probably tell another story instead of an answer—or reply: "I don't know exactly. The story seemed somehow fitting."

In fact, clients hardly ever ask me this question. Should it be expressed, I might interpret it as an indication that the client feels provoked by the telling of a story—be it that it had a moralizing or pedagogical undertone, or that the client felt insecure due to a possibly too abrupt change of perspective, whether the therapist took him seriously.

It is not necessary and probably more harmful than useful to explain the meaning of stories. By turning a metaphor into an allegory and an anecdote into a lesson in this way, possibilities are taken away for the client to interpret the story for himself, and a didactic tone easily creeps in, which can also be perceived as presumptuous. It is also not necessary to return to the original concern (as the supposedly actual problem) of the client after telling a story.

References

Hammel S (2009) Handbuch des therapeutischen Erzählens. Geschichten und Metaphern in Psychotherapie, Kinder- und Familientherapie, Heilkunde, Coaching und Supervision. Klett-Cotta, Stuttgart

Hammel S (2018) Handbook of therapeutic storytelling. Stories and metaphors in psychotherapy, child and family therapy, medical treatment, coaching and supervision. Routledge, London

Hammel S (2022) Hypnosystemische Therapie. Das Handbuch für die Praxis. Klett-Cotta, Stuttgart

Hammel S (2024) Transforming lives with hypnosystemic therapy. A practical guide. Routledge, London

9

Editing Stories—Polishing the Diamond

Trailer

In therapy work, spontaneously improvised stories are often just as effective as carefully crafted narratives. Clients often respond better to authentic communication than to read-out content. Complex stories may require a written elaboration. When editing a story, unnecessary words should be removed, short sentences formed, and abstraction converted into concreteness. Direct speech should be used, evaluations avoided, and surprises not anticipated.

In therapeutic work, it is often necessary to spontaneously improvise stories without any literary claim. The situation does not allow for further refining of the small narrative. Experience says: These stories are therapeutically just as effective as carefully formulated narratives and sometimes more effective, as clients respond better to authentic communication than to read or recited content that does not seem to originate from the therapist's innermost being. It

S. Hammel, *Learning Therapeutic Storytelling*, https://doi.org/10.1007/978-3-662-69110-6_9

is different when the therapist uses the writing of a story to appropriate the story and to address it to the client with particular emphasis. If the therapist does not feel confident enough to recite such a story from memory, he can tell the client: "What you said has still occupied me a lot. I have written down a few words for you. May I recite them to you?" Even if the story is then read out, the client should feel valued and follow the recited with special attention.

For complex stories, a written elaboration may also be necessary to not forget anything and not to miss the punchline. The basic idea of the story could perhaps be compared here to a raw diamond, whose value and beauty are only fully revealed in its polished form.

The Most Important Editing Rules

Here are some rules of thumb for editing stories:

The beginning of a story is often good if it is short and crisp, if it contains a surprise or leads the listener into introspection with a question. The same applies to the end. A surprise, an emotional impulse, a question, a provocation, a slight confusion, or information that puts everything previously said in a new light (punchline, reframing) is advantageous here. Not everything essential should be said, but a transfer into the listener's world should be necessary, an inner search for the meaning of the story in his worldview.

I would comb through the text of the story up to ten times according to the following criteria. Of course, these writing habits automate over time, so that eventually even the first version meets most of the criteria.

1. Put every superfluous word to the test: Does the sentence feel more powerful with this word or without it? The following can probably be omitted:
   - Auxiliary verbs such as: can, could, should, might, etc.
   - Filler words such as: naturally, anytime, in a way, absolutely, as well as, somehow, anyway
   - some binding particles such as: and, also, as well as
2. Form short sentences:
   - separate main clauses strung together with commas by periods
   - transform subordinate clause constructions into main clauses
   - rebuild participle constructions (my reading neighbor, eaten bread) into full sentences
3. Transform abstraction into concreteness:
   - transform words with -ness, -ity, -ty, -ing into verbs (actions)
   - transform foreign words into German words
   - transform attributed properties into actions and perceptions
4. Prefer "and" to "or"
   - check whether "or" can be transformed into "and"
   - check whether "respectively" can be transformed into "or" or "and"
   - use "as well as" in case of too much "and" (and only then)
5. Use direct speech:
   - transform indirect speech into direct speech (quote)
   - formulate thoughts and intentions of people as a quote
   - formulate dialogues

6. Remove evaluations:
   - avoid adjectives with evaluative, especially deroga-tory, character (smart, foolish, stingy, conceited)
   - avoid quotes and action descriptions that suggest lower motives
   - avoid punishment logic
7. Do not anticipate surprises:
   - No hints of later events—or subtly overlooked
   - Signal words for a twist ("suddenly", "surprised") should rather be omitted
   - Surprises come late: at the end of the sentence, the section, the story
8. Insert perceptible and tangible elements (sometimes in contrast to rule 1):
   - Emotions and states of mind make the story tangi-ble: angry, sad, confused
   - Visible, tangible, audible: fiery red, sharp, loud
   - also metaphorically and synaesthetically: a bright bell sound, a harsh blow
9. Avoid logical breaks:
   - the genre rules are adhered to (no scientists in fairy tales, no talking animals in scientific reports). Exceptions must be justified
   - the logical sequence is maintained (not: "I enter. As I press the latch…", but: "I press the latch. As I enter…")
   - vivid details should be shared at the beginning or not at all, but not too late
10. Build protagonists as identification figures
    - Objects, clouds, values ("hope"), are not suitable for identification
    - Describe protagonists as likeable, interesting or neutral
    - adopting the internal perspective can promote identification

11. Transform negative formulations into positive ones
    - in sentences with the structure "not—but" delete the part before the "but"
    - in sentences with "not", write what happens or should happen "instead"
    - Formulations with "un-", "no", "without" etc., if possible, reformulate positively
12. Avoid duplications, triads and longer enumerations
    - Reduce duplications and triads like "fears, troubles and worries" to one term
    - Shorten enumerations to a few exemplary terms or a generic term
    - Reduce several similar sentence constructions ("during… and during") to one
13. Check the order of the parts of the sentence—how does the sentence sound powerful?
    - Instead of: "Calories do not necessarily create energy" rather: "Energy is not a matter of calories"
    - Instead of: "He hid during the day and continued his journey at night" rather: "He hid during the day, he continued his journey at night"
    - Instead of: "He cried: 'Woe!'" rather: "'Woe!' he cried."
14. Avoid platitudes
    - Delete truisms: "It is better to think first and then speak"
    - No worn-out phrases: "Curiosity killed the cat."
    - Instead of: "One morning Gregor got up" (doesn't he always do that?) rather: "Gregor looked out of his cave"

Surely, one does not always need to apply all principles. Nevertheless, it has proven effective to largely follow them and only allow justified deviations.

10

Storytelling in Child and Adolescent Therapy—Gregor, the Dragon

Trailer

Stories with fairy tale elements can be effectively used with children up to primary school age. An example shows how therapy was successfully conducted with an aggressive child. The therapist used a positive identification figure, the dragon, to transform the boy's aggression into positive energy. The involvement of parents and siblings can be beneficial in therapy. They are an additional source of ideas and information, and when the stories told are heard by all involved, favorable interactions usually occur. For teenagers, informative anecdotal and metaphorical stories in their area of interest are often useful.

The stories we tell children should naturally be adapted to their understanding and best fit their interests. Up to primary school age, fables and stories with fairy tale elements can be effectively used with many children. An example...

© The Author(s), under exclusive license to Springer-Verlag GmbH, DE, part of Springer Nature 2024
S. Hammel, *Learning Therapeutic Storytelling*,
https://doi.org/10.1007/978-3-662-69110-6_10

Scratching and Biting

A mother reported that her five-year-old son regularly scratched his older sister until she bled. I asked the mother to bring both children. The older sister surprisingly candidly shared that she deliberately provoked her brother when they were alone so he scratched her until she bled. After this she would run crying to their mother, who punished the brother and comforted her. When asked if this was nice, she answered with a radiant "Yes!". Partners are equal, or in other words: Most people deserve each other. This also applies to conflict partners and siblings. I asked the mother, who followed her daughter's explanations in astonishment, to punish either both children or none at all in conflicts between the siblings in the coming months. This way, she could compensate for the injustice that had happened to the boy and interrupt the conflict pattern.

Stories for Children and their Parents

I told the boy the story of Gregor, the dragon.

Gregor, the Dragon

When Gregor set off one winter morning to play with the animals in the forest, he discovered that none of them wanted anything to do with him. Instead, the fox, the badger, and the bear complained that he had burned, scratched, and bitten their fur. When the dragon then sat lonely and heartbroken in a forest clearing, the owl came to his aid with a plan. He was to tell her quiet dragon stories all night and warm her with his warm dragon neck. In the protection of the darkness, all the animals came one by one to hear his stories and warm themselves on his warm neck. (See Hammel 2009, p. 209 f.)

Already the next week, the mother reported that her children argued less and the boy no longer scratched and bit his sister. The newly discovered ways of reacting apparently proved successful for the boy. Thus, the therapy could be ended after a few hours without the problem returning.

Parents often ask whether they should accompany their children to therapy. Since an additional perspective represents an additional resource for therapy, I usually support this, but suggest that the parents ask their children how they would like it. Almost all younger children and many older ones are glad when they are accompanied by their parents. Often at the beginning, I ask the children: "Should I ask you or your mother what the matter is?" Many children initially find it difficult to talk about their burdens. Some are ashamed of their problem, some are extremely shy, some are masters of repression or pretense, and some lack the linguistic skills to put into words what is bothering them. If a child indicates that his mother should explain the situation, I suggest: "Your mother tells me, and you correct her afterwards if she talks nonsense, okay?" With this, I have conveyed to the child:

- I take you seriously in your autonomy and your right to speak for yourself.
- I do not want to punish, shame, or otherwise emotionally challenge you.
- I am on your side and, if necessary, even against your mother's ideas.

Having one or both parents and possibly also siblings present has another great advantage: The therapist can influence both or all parties involved at the same time to achieve an improvement in the situation. By working from multiple sides, with each side seeing what is happening on the other side, the effect of the therapy is amplified. In the context of therapeutic storytelling, this means: The other family members also hear the story that is told to the child, they experience the child's reaction and relate what happens after the session to it. Of course, we can tell stories that contain a message for all present. We can also address our own stories to the parents, with the children listening and noticing that the parents also need (usually very respectful-discreet) instruction. For the child, this means: "So I'm not the only one to blame for everything! My parents also have to learn something!" Very often, stories that are primarily or mainly addressed to the parents also contain messages for the child's ear.

If the child's life began with a great danger for the little one and sometimes also for the mother, if a child in the family died earlier, or if the mother was in great fear for other reasons, a particularly close bond between mother and child sometimes develops, which, despite all the warmth and security conveyed, can also be burdensome and restrictive for the child's development.

To a very anxious or caring mother, I could tell during the therapy with the child:

Combine Harvesters and Ladybugs

Life can be very hard, and when it is hard, it does not spare small, delicate creatures. Once, a farmer invited me to accompany him on a ride with the combine harvester and to witness how it cut and threshed the wheat in the field in one pass. The combine harvester was quite an old specimen, perhaps from the sixties. I sat high up next to the farmer, who drove the vehicle in long, straight lines across the field. Behind the seat of the driver and passenger was a huge container into which the grain trickled. Thousands, probably millions of wheat grains fell in there. Among them struggled and wriggled—hundreds of ladybugs. What was their perspective? From up there, the grain slid down into the interior of the wagon, where, as the farmer explained to me, it was crushed with large iron bolts to separate the chaff from the wheat. I could see how one ladybug after another disappeared in a funnel of sliding wheat grains. The wheat grains were smaller than the ladybugs. It's unthinkable what was done to the lovable beetles down there. When I later got off the combine harvester, the farmer showed me the container with the threshed wheat. Clean, bright grains, freed from the husks. Here and there and everywhere between them, the ladybugs worked their way up, spread their wings, and flew away!

If it is possible to instill confidence in parents about the resilience of their children, while at the same time appreciating the tenderness that lies in their concern and care, this usually benefits both sides.

Often it is beneficial if it is possible to look at the situation reported by clients with a new perspective of humor and lightness—provided that it does not give the impression that their suffering is to be trivialized.

To a mother who blamed herself for going back to work after the first or second child and the subsequent children then received less attention, I told the following anecdote:

With the Third Child

My mother was talking to a friend about what kind of attention children need and what they get. She said to her: When the first child stumbles and falls, you still ask: "Did you hurt yourself? Everything okay? Nothing broken?" With the third, you just say: "Make sure you don't bleed all over the carpet."

If the "third child" is present, it can be acknowledged how terrible it can be to not be recognized by parents in suffering. At the same time, it can be discussed that less worry does not mean less love, that greater serenity often also means greater freedoms for the younger siblings, and that sometimes older and younger siblings disagree about who had it better—because their position in the family had different advantages and disadvantages for them.

Stories for Teenagers

From the beginning of puberty, it becomes tricky to tell stories with talking animals, fairies, wizards, and the like. If we use genres in conversation with teenagers that are associated with a younger age, the young people may get the impression that we are confusing them with children and not treating them on an equal footing as adults or almost adults. Instead, we can choose metaphors or anecdotes from areas that specifically interest them. The prerequisite is that we are sufficiently informed about the topic and do not appear ingratiating by trying to present ourselves as younger and cooler than is authentically possible for us. Good stories leave enough room for individual transfer to allow for personal interpretations and not to appear instructive.

Example stories can tell how people have overcome problems, weathered crises, and achieved success. Such stories can serve as a model for the clients.

The risk of appearing instructive is most likely when the therapist feels obligated to the concerns of the worried parents and has not thoroughly and credibly explored which goals are important to the teenagers themselves. Some of these goals do not seem very constructive at first glance. Nevertheless, the therapist himself can suggest to the teenager to pursue therapy goals, such as…

- the parents stop annoying them with expectations and lectures,
- the parents increase the pocket money,

- they get better grades and pass the school year with as little work as possible, or
- the classmates stop teasing them.

Once the therapist and the teenage client have agreed on such goals, it can be considered when this works particularly well or particularly badly, how the teenager can stimulate the desired behavior of the parents or persuade the teachers to give better grades, what price one would pay for this in one's own interest, or whether it is more pleasant to leave the situation as it is.

The therapist and the teenager can develop games and experiments to find out how different behaviors affect the behavior of classmates.

To illustrate that such approaches make a significant difference to the teenager's situation, the therapist can tell anecdotes from other teenagers:

> **The Boys at the Bus Stop**
>
> Lena was teased by her classmates for years—bullied, you could say. She had a keen sense of observation. I learned a lot from her. Once, she told me, she was standing at the bus stop in winter. She was wearing a woolen hat with a pom-pom. The boys at the bus stop made a game of grabbing the hat by the pom-pom and trying to pull it off her head. "Stop it!", "That's annoying!", "Stop it, or the pom-pom will come off!" No matter what she said, the boys kept going. At some point, she told me, she decided: The next one who pulls on it, I'll kick as hard as I can in the shin. From that moment on, none of the boys pulled on her hat anymore.

The story illustrates that people react immediately to the inner attitude that someone adopts and to the aura that results from it. To further clarify this, the following story can be used.

Feeling Eighteen Years Old

At times, Lena didn't feel like walking through the pedestrian zone anymore because she constantly ran into classmates who made stupid remarks or showed with various gestures and grimaces that they were making fun of her and looking down on her. Once a thought came to her. She imagined what it would feel like to walk through the city as an eighteen-year-old—even though she was only fourteen. How would she look then? What posture would she have? She noticed: When she walked through the pedestrian zone feeling like she was eighteen, no one made any more stupid gestures, grimaces, or remarks.

Sometimes seminar participants ask me: "How do I continue after a story?" or "What do I do if someone asks me why I'm telling them this story?" My most common answer is: "Stories don't need commentary. Just tell the next story." In fact, the impact of such stories can be enhanced if you present related anecdotes in a series of stories. So we can just continue.

Black Fingernails

Once, Lena and a neighborhood girl painted their fingernails black. Actually, she was more of an eco-intellectual. The black polish was not her style but just a fun action. They removed the nail polish again. Before they were done, the neighborhood girl was called home and took the nail polish and nail polish remover with her. It belonged to her. Lena still had two black fingernails. What the heck, it doesn't matter. When she went to school the next day, she was surprised that none of the classmates teased or taunted her in any way, which usually happened every day. "What's different today?" she asked herself. The only thing she found were the two black fingernails. But could that make such a big difference? The next morning she asked her older brother: "Can you lend me your heavy metal t-shirt and your studded belt?" "Sure. No problem."

> Now the students who used to tease her even deliberately avoided her. The next day she just wore a black t-shirt.

Anecdotes can also be used to invite teenagers to experiment with verbal communication strategies. Here too, I use series of examples:

> **Nonsense Brings Peace**
>
> Some time ago, I told a friend about a man named Erickson. He had the habit of always asking or telling some strange nonsense when someone wanted to accuse him of something. Then the other person was confused for a while and said nothing more. It worked well. When Erickson was training to be a doctor, a professor said to him:
>
> "Erickson, I don't like…" "I don't like the snow either," said Erickson. "What are you talking about?" "About the snow." "Which snow?" "This wonderful miracle—that no two snowflakes are alike." This Erickson believed we "should have some irrelevant remarks ready at all times" (Rosen 1982).
>
> This reminds me of a friend who told me: When I was just coming to you, I had to turn my car around and backed into a garage driveway. The owner of the property was there and yelled and cursed at me terribly. I rolled down the window and said: "I thank you, because you made me sad and I'm very happy about that!"
>
> When I told Lena about it, she said: "On such occasions, I say: 'Buy yourself an umbrella!' It always works. Recently, I silenced the biggest blabbermouth in my class with it."
>
> Another acquaintance explained: "In such cases, I always say: 'Go feed the birds!'"

The therapist can also include biological considerations. The following story can be used, for example, to explain why "the boys at the bus stop" stopped teasing the girl at the mere thought of her kicking them in the shin.

Wolves and Wild Horses

When a pack of wolves is threatened by hunger in a cold Siberian winter, they will not hesitate to attack a herd of wild horses. However, they must proceed with extreme caution. A solid kick with a hoof, and a wolf can be fatally injured. The wolves will circle the wild horse herd for a while and observe them closely. They will notice that some horses tense their muscles, ready to kick out at the first suitable opportunity and, if possible, smash a wolf's skull. Other horses will freeze in fear. The wolves recognize the difference. They do not attack the horses that are about to defend themselves with kicks, but those that cannot defend themselves because they are paralyzed with fear.

In the same way, psychological considerations can be illustrated. The following discussion can illustrate why the measures from the stories "Feeling Eighteen Years Old" and "Black Fingernails" have helped.

The Pull of Change

When you just came in, I greeted you as usual and you greeted me in the same way, everything as usual. If instead I had stepped on your foot as a greeting, you probably wouldn't have managed to behave exactly as usual. And if you had come in with a Tyrolean hat and a gas mask, I wouldn't have managed that either. Different behavior generates different behavior—this also applies to very inconspicuous behavior changes. Even if your voice sounds a bit different, if you dress differently, use different expressions for a while, or do something unusual, the others around you will involuntarily react differently than before. Changed behavior creates a pull that no one can escape. Maybe this is an opportunity. Can I invite you to experiment with this? In this research project, everything is allowed if you follow one rule: behave in a way that you do not annoy, harm or endanger anyone.

Several small scenes, from which whole stories could also be created, are linked here to invite young people to discover the relevance of differentiation. Young people can expand their choices by making observations on questions that can generally be formulated as follows:

- In what ways can I behave differently and what difference does this make for me in the end?
- How can I interpret the same situation differently and what difference does this make for me?
- In what ways do people react differently to me and what is the difference for me?
- What changes in my involuntary experience and behavior and in the reaction of others to me when I integrate fictional elements into the situation experienced in reality in my imagination?

The examples provided here are primarily intended to establish vividness and plausibility and to make young people curious to make their own observations in order to expand their choices and decision-making options in critical situations.

References

Erickson M, Rossi E (1981) Hypnotherapie. Aufbau, Beispiele, Forschungen. Klett-Cotta, Stuttgart

Hammel S (2009) Handbuch des therapeutischen Erzählens. Geschichten und Metaphern in Psychotherapie, Kinder- und Familientherapie, Heilkunde, Coaching und Supervision. Klett-Cotta, München

Hammel S (2016) Loslassen und Leben. Befreiende Geschichten. impress, Mainz

Hammel S (2018) Handbook of therapeutic storytelling. Stories and metaphors in psychotherapy, child and family therapy, medical treatment, coaching and supervision. Routledge, London

Hammel S et al (2018) Wie der Bär zum Tanzen kam. 120 Geschichten für einen gesunden Körper. Reinhardt, München

Lamprecht K (2020) Die Rennschildkröte. 31 therapeutische Geschichten für Kinder. Reinhardt, München

Rosen S (ed) (1982) My Voice Will Go with You. Teaching Tales of Milton H. Erickson. Norton, New York

Short D, Weinspach C (2007) Hoffnung und Resilienz. Therapeutische Strategien von Milton H. Erickson. Carl Auer, Heidelberg

11

Storytelling in Adult Therapy— Like a Pile of Ants

Trailer

Stories and metaphors can be used in therapeutic work with adults in various ways for different stressors, such as bullying, burnout, difficult family relationships, and traumas. In experiences of overload, such as grief or separation, a metaphor can help find meaning in life. In experiences of inner turmoil, aimlessness, or loss of identity, stories can help find a sense of purpose, generate hope, and build something new after the old life has been destroyed. The metaphors told are often valued by clients more than concrete tips and instructions.

In this chapter, I provide some examples of how stories can be used in therapeutic work with adults.

In the professional field, situations of bullying, unclear and contradictory communication, burnout, and overwork lead people to therapy—although in the latter case

© The Author(s), under exclusive license to Springer-Verlag
GmbH, DE, part of Springer Nature 2024
S. Hammel, *Learning Therapeutic Storytelling*,
https://doi.org/10.1007/978-3-662-69110-6_11

it is not said whether the demanding behavior of superiors, colleagues, and customers or the unsuccessful demarcation of the client contributes more to the stress. In stressors presented under the term "burnout", I see less the amount of work than the constant working against inner resistances, caused perhaps by value conflicts, in the foreground.

To some, I tell about the "Pareto Principle":

Autopilot

Have you heard that with 20% of the energy needed for a 100% result, you can achieve 80% of the desired result? If you set the overall goal well below world record level, sometimes with 10% of the energy you can achieve 90% of the result or with 5% energy expenditure 95%? I would like to invite you to do an experiment. I would like to ask you to do only as much as necessary at your work for three days to avoid disasters, just the bare minimum—as if with the strength of your little finger. You already have your routine, your rituals. Fly on autopilot for three days and only make minimal adjustments when special circumstances arise that require intervention. Is it okay to try this for three days?

Some people, who have achieved and exceeded their goals with a lot of effort through many crises, persist in striving, even when the initially critical situation no longer exists. Some, who had to save themselves in their youth from a world of neglect (see for example the story "Marie" in Chap. 13), who had to free themselves from debts or who were raised to deny themselves and achieve a lot with little praise, continue in this way until they end up in a realm of exhaustion and disappointment. To them, I tell something like the following…

Motor Glider

Imagine you are piloting a glider. In the beginning, you needed a motor plane that pulled your plane up with some energy expenditure. Then you press a button, it clicks, the line releases you and you continue to fly alone. You float in the air, you don't even need energy. The updraft carries you upwards.

But perhaps your plane is a motor glider. These planes don't need anyone to pull them up, they can do it on their own. After that, the principle is the same. You turn off the engine and float in wonderful silence. You can also leave the engine on and continue flying with speed and fuel consumption. But perhaps you would like to experience that your plane also flies safely with the engine off. And if there really is a special reason, turbulence in the air or any emergency, then you can turn the engine back on.

People who are regularly exposed to stressful situations at work, perhaps even personal attacks, I sometimes tell the metaphor…

Laser Pointer Disc

In air traffic, there is the problem that people repeatedly try to dazzle pilots from the ground with laser pointers. This is unpleasant and potentially harmful to the pilots' health, and of course also dangerous for the passengers. Some time ago, someone developed a method to counter this danger. A layer of transparent liquid crystal is applied between the double glass panes of the cockpit. The normally clear substance turns black when a laser beam hits it, but only exactly where the beam shines and only as long as it is there. As soon as the beam is gone, the pane is completely clear again within thousandths of a second.

Imagine you have such a special glass pane around you that reacts to insults. Within thousandths of a second, much faster than an offensive word can reach your consciousness, it turns color and shields you against it. I would like to ask your brain to set up such a preconscious protection mechanism. What do you think, is that okay for your brain?

Of course, such a metaphor can also be used in the context of difficult family relationships, for children and adolescents with problems in the classroom, or for traumatized people who need to protect themselves against sudden overload.

When it comes to bullying or other forms of dehumanizing working conditions, people often describe uncertainty about their identity. Experiences of depersonalization can also be caused by isolation, for example by external seclusion as an individual or in a small group that does not convey a sense of protection (such as accommodation in a barracks, a prison, or a boarding school).

License Plates

When I came back from shopping, I was surprised to see my car surrounded by people—young men with a foreign appearance. I wondered what they wanted. Regardless, as I approached my car, they stepped aside. I got into my car and drove home. "Maybe you should get new license plates," a friend said the next day, looking at my car. "Why?" "It has Romanian license plates."

Wrong labels can cause confusion—this also applies to labels that are attached to people. This story signals to clients who are disturbed in their identity by negative attributions or poor treatment at work or in the family: "It's not you who are wrong, but there's something wrong with the label that was attached to you."

Sometimes it can also be seen that it is not (or not only) the fellow human beings who attach a wrong label to the client, but that our clients label their fellow human beings, such as their colleagues, inappropriately. One can combine a little psychoeducation with a short case example or a metaphor…

Thirteen

I'm not a fan of Sigmund Freud, but some of what he says is very useful. For example, the thing about transferences and countertransferences.

Do you have problems with your superiors, with colleagues, with customers, cooperation partners or subordinates?

Does your boss or your boss behave towards you like someone from your family of origin? Like your father or your mother or someone else? Is there a colleague who treats you like your big brother or a colleague who behaves like your little sister? Could it also be that you behave towards these people as you do towards your parents and siblings?

I asked a client how many people at her workplace she found "difficult". She counted: "Thirteen." I asked how many people her family of origin consisted of. "Thirteen." And after a short pause, she added, surprised and almost frightened: "That's amazing: I can exactly say who from the people at my workplace is who from my siblings, parents and grandparents."

Of course, this is an invitation to the current client to do the same experiment with the people in their own work field. It's amazing how many people make similar discoveries. The therapy can be continued with a metaphor…

Slides

Surely you know them: There are still these overhead projectors, with which you can project different slides one after the other onto the wall. If you put any slides on the projector at the same time, you see everything at once, but understand nothing because the information on the slides does not belong together. If you put two such slides on one after the other, you can read all the information well.

Imagine the image of your boss like two projected slides overlapping on the wall. If it makes sense to you to slide one slide to the left—who could that be? Your father? Your big brother? Someone else? And if you slide someone to the left out of the picture of your boss and your most important colleagues—would there also be family members? Slide all family members to the left into a pile and all members of your workplace to the right. Have you sorted them? If you look again at the team at work—what is different when you see them now?

Overload experiences can also lead to a sense of inner disruption, aimlessness and disorientation. This includes experiences of grief or separation, the sudden loss of health, the workplace, public reputation in society or even moving to a different cultural region. The following metaphor provides an example of how such experiences can be filled with a sense of purpose.

Purposeful as a Pile of Ants

Have you ever looked at an anthill? Again and again, you can see how the animals run back and forth on it, sometimes to the right, then to the left, then forward, only to possibly turn around and run in the opposite direction. If you look at the individual ants on such a pile, it seems to be complete chaos. But if you look at the pile as a whole, you can only marvel at how purposefully everything is obviously laid out. How can it be that the ants, with their seemingly chaotic back and forth, end up being so well organized? Obviously, these are search movements they are making. They test various possibilities of where they can go, then they choose the best one. Immediately afterwards, they test several possibilities again and again and again. The animals' movements are quite wild when someone has damaged the anthill. Frantically and completely chaotically, without sense and reason, the animals seem to wander around, and yet—in a relatively short time, the ants have rebuilt their pile.

Perhaps your inner life seems similarly chaotic to you. It won't look like it at first glance, but maybe it's allowed for me to say: What may now seem completely disorderly, aimless and unstructured to you are search movements of your soul. Because this is happening according to an unconscious program, it appears crazy and meaningless to conscious thinking. In reality, your inner self is busy rebuilding your identity, which has suffered a blow due to a severe loss. In many places, it will be different than before, but presumably better in view of the new situation.

If the client comes to therapy for a long time after such a catastrophic experience, the focus will be more on looking forward: How can I build something new after the old life was destroyed? To generate confidence here, anecdotes and metaphors are often more valuable than concrete tips and instructions, which may work—or not. Anecdotes and metaphors to invite people to a hopeful look forward—an example for each of the two variants:

The Last Child

"I've heard 'That was my last child!' at many births," a midwife told me. "A year later, the same woman is back. When I remind her of her words from the previous year, she grins a little: 'Did I say that? Well, anyway, I'm here now!'"

The next story can be used to encourage people looking for a partner not to be discouraged by loneliness and disappointments, or to encourage people in a professional crisis to reorient themselves professionally.

Web Spiders, Running Spiders, Jumping Spiders

Some people don't like spiders. But you can learn so much from them. Spiders are super interesting. May I tell you something about them?

There are web spiders and running spiders. The two have fundamentally different lifestyles. The former build a web of spider threads, then wait until an animal lands in their trap all by itself. The latter run so fast that they hunt their prey.

There is a third kind, the jumping spiders. They jump like a flea into the air and surprisingly drop from above onto their prey.

If I imagine that you were looking for a juicy piece of prey, (forgive me for saying so,) what would be the most suitable method for you?

The potential uses of stories in psychotherapy are so diverse that any number of additional examples could be added here. Instead of extending the list, reference is made to the relevant literature (Casula 2017; Hammel 2009, 2016a, b, 2018, 2023; Hammond 1990; Trenkle 2016; Watzlawick 1983; Rosen 2009 et al.).

References

Casula C (2017) Gärtner, Prinzessinnen, Stachelschweine. Metaphern und Geschichten für die persönliche und berufliche Entwicklung. Carl Auer, Heidelberg

Hammel S (2009) Handbuch des therapeutischen Erzählens. Geschichten und Metaphern in Psychotherapie, Kinder- und

Familientherapie, Heilkunde, Coaching und Supervision. Klett-Cotta, Stuttgart

Hammel S (2016a) Loslassen und Leben. Befreiende Geschichten. impress, Mainz

Hammel S (2016b) Alles neu gerahmt! Psychische Symptome in ungewöhnlicher Perspektive. München, Reinhardt

Hammel S (2018) Handbook of therapeutic storytelling. Stories and metaphors in psychotherapy, child and family therapy, medical tratment, coaching and supervision. Routledge, London

Hammel S et al (2023) Wie das Nashorn Freiheit fand. 120 Geschichten zum Umgang mit Krisen. Reinhard, München

Hammond C (ed) (1990) Handbook of hypnotic suggestions and metaphors. Norton, New York

Rosen S (ed) (1982) My Voice Will Go with You. Teaching Tales of Milton H. Erickson. Norton, New York

Trenkle B (2016) 3 Bonbons für 5 Jungs. Strategische Hypnotherapie in Fallbeispielen und Geschichten. Carl Auer, Heidelberg

Watzlawick P (1983) The Situation Is Hopeless, But Not Serious. The Pursuit of Unhappiness. Norton, New York

12

Storytelling in Medicine—Rowing Upwards

Trailer

Examples are used to demonstrate how stories can be used in medicine. In our culture, we often separate body and mind, but research shows their inseparable connection. Physical complaints can be caused by psychological stress and vice versa. Case studies can be used to show how mental anesthesia without trance is achieved and how we can stimulate the organism for self-regulation. Metaphors can explain the task of medicine and improve the patients' willingness to cooperate (compliance). The body can be stimulated by metaphors to perform tasks such as the identification and disposal of dysfunctional cells.

Influenced by Platonic philosophy, we are accustomed in our culture to distinguish between body and mind (or Aristotelian between body, mind, and spirit). However, for several decades, research in psychosomatics and psychoneuroimmunology, neuroscience, and epigenetics has

© The Author(s), under exclusive license to Springer-Verlag
GmbH, DE, part of Springer Nature 2024
S. Hammel, *Learning Therapeutic Storytelling*,
https://doi.org/10.1007/978-3-662-69110-6_12

increasingly revealed that the body, our emotions, our memories, expectations, and other thoughts are not at all separable, but are interconnected and linked in every way to form a complete unity. Chinese and Ayurvedic medicine and the approaches of indigenous peoples do not know a body-mind separation and accordingly no distinction between physical and psychotherapeutic treatment forms.

In fact, new possibilities open up when we tentatively assume that physical disorders result from biographical burdens and that they can be fundamentally resolved by lifting remembered and reactivatable psychobiological stress reactions (for example in the context of trauma therapeutic work). Stories are told about hypnotherapeutic approaches that have proven themselves in casual conversation without explicit trance induction or other procedures that can be integrated into the working day without much additional time. The recipients of such case studies are either the patients themselves or the professional helpers. An increased self-responsibility of patients for their health is to be welcomed, provided that self-responsible measures for symptom reduction do not make medical diagnostics superfluous.

Rheumatic Complaints

"Hello. I am a hospital chaplain and would like to inquire how you are doing." "I came here this morning. I had a severe rheumatic flare-up. I have severe pain," said the man.

He sat tense on the edge of the bed and looked at me. "And you are probably here so that the doctors can magic away your pain a bit…?", I asked him.

"Can you do that? Can you magic away my pain?"

Was the man hard of hearing? I hadn't said that at all!

I could have replied "No", but that felt like a lie. "Yes" didn't quite fit either. What should I answer? It occurred to me that Jesus had not turned away those who asked for a miracle. "No work without a contract" is what they say in systemic therapy, but this was a contract, and more like a desperate appeal…

"Let's see what your body can do for you. May I borrow your arm for a moment? Thank you… Imagine you were a tree and this arm was a branch… What kind of tree are you?" "An elm." "Very nice! A great, rare tree! Can you imagine that such an elm feels nothing at all?" "Yes, yes…" There's a lot of snow on the branch, it's been there for many hours. If there was snow on your arm for hours, you wouldn't feel anything either, would you?" "That's true…" "So the arm has been full of snow for hours, or the branch, if you look at it that way. What is currently the most numb area of your arm?" "There at the wrist." "And if the numb feeling at the wrist were a light, what color would it be?" "Yellow." "Let this beautiful yellow light shine brighter and brighter, then spread it all over your arm, and then let it travel through your chest and back to the other side. You can also touch your bright hand with the not so bright one, then it goes even faster… you're doing that very well. Let the light travel up to the top of your head and down your back. You can also imagine how melting snow runs down your back and especially to the places that need it most. Which would those be?" "The knees." "Let the light and the snow go there especially, and when it's good there, what's next?" "The neck." "There now too!" We talked like this for a while. "I see that you're swinging your legs like a little boy on a swing. You look quite cheerful! How are you?" "That can't be! How is that possible? I don't have any pain anymore…"

"The fact that it can be, you notice by the fact that it is so. Say a nice greeting to your body, this is here to stay, and if any remnant of the previous state would come by again to see if you might need that from before again, then I would like to ask you to sit down, swing your legs and do the things with your body that we did today…"

Case stories like this can be used in supervision to illustrate how mental anesthesia can be achieved without trance induction by utilizing and gradually shifting expectations. (For more details, see Hammel 2009, p. 70 ff., 2011, p. 53 ff., 2014, p. 74 ff.)

Common Cold

"I don't know if I'll still be here tomorrow," a seminar participant announced. "I have a pretty severe infection." "What symptoms do you have?" "A blocked nose, a dry cough that doesn't produce anything, headaches, sore throat, body aches, I'm totally weak. I think I also have a fever." "It's strange: What good is a blocked nose? No bacteria are disposed of, and the air that could otherwise contribute to healing also doesn't get in. This cough also does nothing to rid the body of germs and pollutants. And the pain and fever consume so much energy that the body could otherwise use for healing, that one can also ask: What good is that. But it could be: If you didn't have the symptoms, you would demand full work performance from yourself, do sports, walk around thinly dressed in the cold and other things that are not good for your body. Your body doesn't need the symptoms for healing. It only produces them so that you don't do this nonsense that would hinder healing. You could propose a deal to your body: 'Please reduce the symptoms as far as possible, preferably to zero: Reduce the nasal congestion, reduce the cough more and more, the sore throat as well, the headaches too, the body aches as well, the fever and the inflammations as well, and instead of the weakness spread energy and alertness in me. In return, I will spare you just as I would have spared you if you had kept the symptoms, and even better. If I do that, please reduce the symptoms all the way down to zero. If I don't stick to it, you can increase them again'. What do you think, is your body okay with the deal?" "I think my body says 'Yes'. I'm already feeling better." "How do you notice that your body says 'Yes'?" "The headache and the body aches are less, I feel less weak and feverish, and the left nostril is free." "You also haven't coughed lately, your muscles seem more relaxed and you seem to breathe more freely. Your voice also sounds stronger and more resonant. Ask your body if it will also free up the right nostril for you on a trial basis." "Yes, that's getting

> freer now." "Tell your body, he's doing great, he should continue to expand this and you'll remember to spare him. Do you think your body agrees with that?" "He's already on it."

In the same way, personal experiences can be used as examples to show how the organism can be stimulated to self-regulate.

> **Scalding**
>
> I held the tea cup in my right hand, the thermos flask with hot water in my left. I didn't know that the lid was only loosely on the can. Seconds later, the boiling water poured over my hand. "Let all cells live, preserve all that can make it," I said to my hand, while cool water from the tap ran over it. "You've survived. I know you're very shocked now, but you can let go now, like a child that I hold in my arms and comfort. You don't need to do anything, I'll take care of you. We'll go to the doctor soon, who will take care of you. Relax and let go. I'll take care of you."
>
> What remained? No pain, hardly any itching and a surprisingly small blister.

What is described here is an intervention in the style of greetings to the organism (Hammel 2017, 2020, 2022, p. 271 ff., 2024) The next example of helpful handling of one's own pain is a little more complex, but still so manageable that it can be easily passed on to patients. An overlooking of symptoms due to self-therapeutic methods is rather not to be expected: Pain that has a more far-reaching meaning as an important, medically relevant signal will not disappear permanently in such a way. Nevertheless, it makes sense to encourage patients to find a balance, so that they help themselves where possible, but do not overlook persistent symptoms with permanent self-efforts.

Sacroiliac Joint Pain

"What happened to your hip pain that you had at the seminar recently," a training participant asked me. "Which hip pain?" "Didn't you have pain?" "Ah, right, the sacroiliac joint pain." I sat down at the time and asked myself: If I could turn it into an emotion, which one would it be? And can I feel it too?—Yes. I became sad. It was a deep sadness that I hadn't been aware of before.

I asked myself: Can I feel this feeling even more clearly and maybe get an idea of what I'm sad about?—Yes, I knew what I was sad about.

And if I now feel into my hip, how is it now?—Much better, but something is still left.

If I could transform this remaining feeling into an emotion, which one would it be?—Anger…!

Can I really feel this anger emotionally?—Yes, of course…

And if the rest of the rest, which is still there now, were a feeling?—I could feel fear and powerlessness.

Then I felt again. Almost nothing was left of the previous pain. The day after next, it had completely disappeared.

The story is an invitation to listeners to try something similar with their symptoms—and to therapists to test this approach with patients. The approach may seem too simple to be effective, but the results—not only with pain, but also with a variety of other symptoms—are extremely astonishing.

Instead of using case histories, we can also explain a medical situation in other pragmatic and illustrative ways.

I explain to patients with cancer that their body produces cancer cells every day, and that it carefully eliminates these every day. A problem only arises when the body cannot keep up with the removal of damaged cells as quickly as they occur. If the body is behind in cleaning up for a while, it becomes all the more important to tackle this task decisively. This is where the help of specialists is needed, who support the body in its task until it can take over its task well on its own again.

Metaphors can be used to illustrate the task at hand.

Cancer Therapy

I imagine a cancer disease as if I am drifting in a river with my boat. If I want to go upstream, I have to row faster upwards than the water flows downwards. To move forward as quickly and safely as possible, I put together a team of several rowers who take me where I want to go.

When I have reached my destination, I do not say "Done!", let go of everything and drift relieved, but either I row a little further with little effort to maintain my position in the river, or I tie my boat well and check from time to time that it is in good condition and tied as desired.

Metaphors can not only be used to explain the task of medicine and improve the willingness of patients to cooperate (compliance), they can also be used to stimulate the body to implement its very own task—in this case the identification and disposal of dysfunctional cells.

Tumor

In my garden, I have an apple tree. Every autumn, I harvest the fruits and store them in my garage. It is important that I regularly pick out the rotten apples. At the first signs of a rotten spot, I take them out. I collect them in a box and take them to the compost. I have noticed that mice, hedgehogs, and various garden birds feast on them there and eat them up over time. Once, a load of walnuts rotted on me. I also took them to the compost. In winter, there was a lot of snow, and I was hardly in the garden. When I walked through the garden again in the spring, I noticed that the walnuts were no longer on the compost. Under the fruit trees, however, some distance from the compost

> heap, there were large amounts of empty walnut shells.
> The squirrels had carried the nuts up the trees, eaten them
> there, and simply dropped the empty shells at the end.

The following case history can be told to clients to generate plausibility for the assumption that the described dynamics can also arise in them, combined with a corresponding task for self-observation. It can also be used in training and supervision, e.g., to illustrate the effect of auto-suggestion and foreign suggestion or the sensible use of observation tasks in medical therapy.

Alopecia Areata

"I have another concern," said a young client towards the end of the therapy session. "I suffer from alopecia areata. Can you do something about it?" "I have the impression that we have worked very successfully together today," I replied, "and that the alopecia areata, as you call it, has a lot to do with this issue, which I think we have successfully dealt with. Therefore, I wonder whether you still have alopecia areata at all, or whether it is possible that it has started to stop today. We have not yet visited the future. All we know is that you have had alopecia areata *so far*. Perhaps you now have circular hair growth, and just as the hair previously fell out from the inside out, it may now be growing back from the outside in. You cannot consciously know this, but it cannot be disproved either. Therefore, I would like to ask you to simply observe whether my assumption is correct that your scalp has started to produce circular hair growth today. When we see each other next time, I ask you to report to me about it." The client came back two weeks later and reported that the hair had regrown at the said spot.

The next story illustrates how the imagination of technical devices and their functions can be used to stimulate the organism to better regulate body functions. Formally considered, the static metaphor of the story "Filter Systems" in Chap. 2 is similar.

Overheating

A seminar participant who was significantly overweight due to illness asked me during a hot summer weather phase what she could do to not suffer so much from the heat. If the weather stayed like this, she was concerned whether she could continue to participate in the seminar. I said, "Last week, heating technicians installed a heat exchanger in my house. It's a fascinating thing. My father told me about it. He taught refrigeration technology at the university of applied sciences. The principle has been known since the 19th century, but we really started using these types of devices when we got electrical power in our homes. On one side of the device, the air is cooled, on the other, it is heated. The whole thing works via circulating water, which absorbs the heat on one side and releases it on the other. Refrigerators work like this: cold inside, warm outside. Air conditioners do the same: the rooms inside are cooled, the world outside is heated. My heating engineer explained to me that there is a temperature range where the heat exchanger works particularly well. Above and below that, the device also works, it just needs more electricity. Your body also has a heat exchanger. Tell it to see how it can adjust the circulation pump to better transfer the heat from inside to outside. The participant was satisfied with this answer, actively participated in the seminar, and otherwise seemed to cope well with the temperature from then on."

I remember a similar, in some ways reversed, experience from my training period.

Undercooling

During our hypnotherapy training, we were supposed to practice trance inductions. It was winter, and the heating in the seminar building worked, if at all, very inadequately.

> We were miserably cold. "I wish for a warming hypnosis," said a small group participant. We others agreed and out-did each other with suggestions of turned-up heaters and blazing bonfires. "There's one thing I didn't understand," I asked the hypnotized person after the exercise. "Why did you keep rubbing your hands while we were talking?" "I was sweating so much. It was already too hot, and you kept talking."

The examples mentioned are representative of countless variations on how we can work with stories in medicine, nursing, and various forms of body therapy.

Other areas of application include—to name just a few examples—allergy therapy (Hammel 2017, p. 116 ff.; Unterberger et al. 2014, p. 23 ff., Sellam 2006, p. 37 ff.; Abraham 1990, p. 265 f.) tinnitus therapy (Hammel 2009; Erickson 1990; Steinriede 2002, 2009), wart treatment (Hammel 2009, p. 64; Hammel 2022, p. 84 f.; Hammel 2024; Hammond 1990, p. 223 ff.; Höller, Béguelin 2009) and blood clotting (Bishay et al. 1990; Olness, Cohen 2001, p. 278 ff., 320, Stoler, 1990a, b, c, p. 286, 291).

References

Abraham H (1990) Suggestions for prevention of seasonal allergies. In: Hammond (Hrsg) Handbook of hypnotic suggestions and metaphors. Norton, New York, S. 265f

Bishay E et al (1990) Suggestions for control of upper gastrointestinal hemmorrhage. In: Hammond (Hrsg) Handbook of hypnotic suggestions and metaphors. Norton, New York, S. 245f

Erickson M (1990) Erickson's Metaphor with Tinnitus. In: Hammond (ed) Handbook of hypnotic suggestions and metaphors. Norton, New York, S 266

Hammel S (2006) Der Grashalm in der Wüste. Metaphern und Geschichten in Beratung, Therapie und Seelsorge. impress, Mainz

Hammel (2009) Tinitustherapie durch Hypnose. Der Heidelberger Pilotversuch. Musica Sacra 04/09 223ff

Hammel S (2011) Handbuch der therapeutischen Utilisation. Vom Nutzen des Unnützen in Psychotherapie, Kinder- und Familientherapie, Heilkunde und Beratung. Klett-Cotta, Stuttgart

Hammel S (2012) The Blade of grass in the Desert. Storytelling: Forgotten medicine for healing the soul. A story of 100 stories for counselling and therapy. impress, Mainz

Hammel S (2014) Therapie zwischen den Zeilen. Das ungesagt Gesagte in Psychotherapie, Beratung und Heilkunde. Klett-Cotta, Stuttgart

Hammel S (2017) Grüßen Sie Ihre Seele. Therapeutische Interventionen in drei Sätzen. Klett-Cotta, Stuttgart

Hammel S (2019) Therapeutic interventions in three sentences reshaping Ericksonian Hypnotherapy by talking to the Brain and Body, Routledge, London

Hammel S (2020) Therapeutic Interventions in Three Sentences. Reshaping Ericksonian Hypnotherapy by talking to the Brain and Body. Routledge, London

Hammel S (2022) Hypnosystemische Therapie. Das Handbuch für die Praxis. Klett-Cotta, Stuttgart

Hammel S (2024) Transforming lives with hypnosystemic therapy. A practical guide. Routledge, London

Hammel S et al (2018) Wie der Bär zum Tanzen kam. 120 Geschichten für einen gesunden Körper. Reinhardt, München

Hammond (1990) Handbook of Hypnotic Suggestions and Metaphors. Norton, New York

Höller J, Béguelin C (1990) Warzen. In: Revenstorf P (Hrsg) Hypnose in Psychotherapie, Psychosomatik und Medizin. Manual für die Praxis. Springer Medizin, Heidelberg

Sellam S (2006) Les allergies. C'est plus simple qu'on le pense. Bérangel, Montreuil-Bonnin

Steinriede R (2002) Medizinische Hypnose bei Tinnitus und Hörsturz. Carl Auer, Heidelberg

Steinriede R (2009) Tinnitus und Hörsturz. In: Revenstorf P (Hrsg) Hypnose in Psychotherapie, Psychosomatik und Medizin. Manual für die Praxis. Springer Medizin, Heidelberg

Stoler D (1990) Childbirth script. In: Hammond (Hrsg) Handbook of hypnotic suggestions and metaphors. Norton, New York, 286 ff.

Unterberger G et al (2014) Allergien mental behandeln. Damit Geist und Körper wieder angemessen reagieren können – Modelle und Strategien angewandter Psychoneuroimmunologie. Psymed, Bargteheide

13

Storytelling in Therapy Training and Supervision—Matryoshka

Trailer

Therapeutic stories can be used not only in therapy, but also in training and supervision. They help to illustrate complex relationships and clarify goals. Metaphors can be used to stimulate the organism for self-regulation and to test new perspectives and behaviors. Circular causalities are taken into account, and self-fulfilling prophecies can play a role. Therapists should adapt their methods to the individual needs of the clients to achieve successful results. For example, stories of liberation can be used to dissolve destructive dependencies.

Of course, therapeutic stories can be used not only in therapy itself, but also in therapy training and supervision. They help to illustrate relationships in a memorable way. For example…

Goal and Task Clarification

In systemic and hypnosystemic work, we begin therapy, each session, and each new section of a session with goal and task clarification.

Classically systemic therapists engage with different questioning techniques to ensure that their clients provide them with a positively formulated, concrete, vivid, and achievable goal as a basis for their joint work. When asked what clients want to achieve, they often do not share the goal of their desires, but explain what they no longer want. Apparently, it is easier for them to communicate what should stop than what they wish for instead. To illustrate the difficulties associated with this, I tell training participants, supervisees, and sometimes clients the following.

> **Ticket Counter**
>
> When you go to the train station and want to buy a train ticket at the counter, the man at the counter asks you where you want to go.
>
> If you say: "Away from here!", he replies: "We don't have 'away' here! You have to tell me where you want to go!" If you insist that you just want to get away and don't tell him where you want to go, he won't sell you a ticket. "I have other customers here. Come back when you know where you want to go!"
>
> The unconscious is a ticket seller. If you only tell it what you don't want and not what you want instead, the likelihood is high that you will stay where you are.

When working *hypnosystemically*, the main addressee of therapy is not the conscious, but the unconscious, i.e., the entire organism with its broader possibilities.

Travel Agency

When you go to a travel agency, it's a bit different. When you stand at the counter and say: "I want to get away from here!" then the woman (or man) says to you:

"You've come to the right place! We have some very affordable offers right now. Let's take a look...!"

In Hypnosystemic Therapy, it's okay to first make offers that are incompatible with the unwanted status quo, represent a felt, approximate opposite of the previous, and then see what the client chooses.

The therapist can also make offers of a possible goal setting and ask the client if pursuing such goals is in her interest. An illustration can be a story from Homer's Odyssey.

Scylla and Charybdis

A famous sailor once had to sail through the Strait of Messina. It's a narrow sea passage, and on each shore of the narrow passage lived a monster. On one side lived Scylla, with six heads and three rows of teeth in each jaw. Scylla devoured anyone who came near her, skin and all. On the other side lived Charybdis. He sucked in all the seawater three times a day and then burped it out again. Any ship that got caught in his pull was lost.

But the sailor made it, he steered his ship between the sea monsters, to the other side, to the safe home port.

I see our therapy a bit similar. We want to get out of the pull of depression and the zone of numbness. But depression has the function of freezing something that once hurt very much: homelessness, grief, loneliness, powerlessness, or anger.

We don't want to go there either. Our goal could be to keep the ship in the zone in between, so that you can feel yourself again, physically and emotionally, and yet nothing ever gets out of hand. Is that in your interest?

Initiation of Helpful Experience without Problem

Next, the therapist can find out with the client how he feels when involuntary instances of his body dissociate the unwanted symptomatic experience: "If you imagine that the one who drinks to numb himself steps out of you and stands over there, where does he stand? How does he look? How does he stand there? And what difference does it make for you if he stands there? What is different about you now when you feel inside yourself?" (Hammel 2019, p. 29 f., 2022, p. 264 ff; Hammel 2024.)

The dynamics of a therapy with such interventions can again be illustrated with stories.

> **Matryoshka**
>
> When you remove a shell from a Russian Matryoshka figure, you find the next one behind it, and the next one behind that, which is slightly smaller, and yet another one, even smaller. Thus, you find the next one behind each shell.
>
> You remove the shells in the reverse order in which they were assembled. Similarly, in therapy, when you work with the symptoms that are apparent and look at what comes next. The physical, emotional, and social adaptation strategies that manifest as symptoms usually emerged in the reverse order in which they appear to you in therapy.
>
> When you look at such a Matryoshka shell, you find that it consists of two layers. On the outside is a hard, perhaps colorful lacquer, and inside is soft, vulnerable wood. It is often the same with the symptoms you are working on. First, you always see rigidity or numbness or something colorful that distracts. When you set that aside, pain appears behind it: loneliness, powerlessness, grief, overwhelming fear, or disgust.

Sometimes as a therapist, you have an inkling of what will emerge next in a conversation with a client, and sometimes you are surprised.

Being Open to Surprises

It seems important to me to be curious on the one hand, whether your own hypotheses and forecasts are confirmed, and on the other hand, to be open to the possibility that something completely different turns out to be accurate or effective instead.

> **The Search for the Hoopoe**
>
> Many years ago, I visited a friend in Poland. I asked him if there were hoopoes in his area. I wanted so much to see such a bird. "Did you come here for that?" The friend laughed a lot about my wish. Seeing a hoopoe was as ordinary for him as it was for me to look at a crow or magpie. He told me a place where I could go, where he thought I would see many hoopoes. I spent most of the day at the indicated place, found not a single hoopoe, and instead saw a beautiful kingfisher. Many years later, I went to a beach in Spain where I expected to see seagulls. There weren't many of them. Instead, I encountered a hoopoe.

Expecting Circular Processes

Coming from systemic work, hypnosystemic therapy usually does not expect linear, but circular causalities. What is perceived as a problem is usually something that recurs persistently. And what recurs stably in a system is maintained by processes between different system elements or subsystems, which can be described in cycles.

However, we often only perceive half of such a cycle, which is why we expect a linear correlation. For example, a client might tell us about his addiction, but not about a professional situation in which he is very successful, but regularly works until he is exhausted and frustrated—and also not about the fact that out of shame for losing control, after an evening when he has comforted himself with alcohol, he works even more intensively and effectively the next day.

We may only learn that his wife has wanted to separate from her husband for a long time because of his alcohol consumption, but not that he has been consuming alcohol for years because his wife wants to separate from him and in doing so, the childhood drama of his adoption is reactivated again and again.

We may only learn that his wife's depression keeps her awake at night, but not that this insomnia contributes to maintaining the depression.

Escalators

When I was four, I wondered where the escalators go when they disappear back into the ground at the end of my ride. How long might they be? Where did they start? Where did they end? Were they infinite? It was very interesting for me when my older brother explained to me that the steps of the escalator run back underground, right back to where I see them coming out of the ground again.

A particular type of circular processes is often referred to as a self-fulfilling prophecy. Of course, not every self-fulfilling prophecy has to be part of a circular process and not every prophecy has to come true, however, there is a dynamic that ensures that prophecies that come true easily lead into circular processes.

The Cycle of Memory and Expectation

When I walk on black ice and fear that I might fall, my muscles tense up and become inflexible. This increases the likelihood that I will fall. If I intuitively notice how insecure I am moving on the ice, my insecurity grows, my muscles tense up even more, become even more inflexible, and the probability that I will fall increases further, until I might actually fall.

If I expect my boss to judge me and possibly treat me poorly, I will watch him suspiciously. I probably try to hide my mistrust, but my behavior may appear even less authentic, open, and accommodating, in short, even less trustworthy. It is quite possible that my boss then judges me and possibly treats me poorly.

If I expect a pill to help me, it may work, even if it is a placebo and contains no active ingredient. And if I expect to get the side effects listed in the package insert, that can also happen, even if it is a placebo. (This is called the "nocebo effect".)

Thus, what I expect becomes what I experience. And what I experience becomes what I remember. And what I remember becomes what I expect. After three or four rounds in which expectation has become experience, experience has become memory, and memory has become expectation, I speak of experience. Eventually, I have collected a lot of experience and say: "So much experience cannot be deceptive."

Once a pattern in a person's or group's behavior has been established, it continues until a special reason arises that makes it necessary to change it. This is usually the case when something changes in the context in which the pattern is shown. Such context changes often arise from cumulative changes that result from the pattern itself. For example, someone might quit smoking after having a lung carcinoma removed that was caused by smoking. The pattern can also be interrupted by external influences that have nothing to do with the self-stabilizing system, but are associated with it. For example, a woman might quit smoking because she has become pregnant.

What Proves Itself, what is Perceived and Believed, Remains

The fact that established patterns continue stably as long as nothing interrupts them can be illustrated in training and supervision with various stories.

1492

Do you know what happened in 1492? "Yes," you say, "America was discovered." But in 1492 there was another event without which Columbus would never have embarked on his journey. That year, after a hundred years of Spanish conquest campaigns, the last emirate in Europe fell with Granada. The Reconquista was over, and the Spaniards had time and money to turn to something new. But when they arrived in America, they did not behave as if peace had now been established. They continued the war by wresting territory from the so-called heathens, with murder and looting. Yet the indigenous people had done nothing to them. Why did they do that? They were used to it and it had proven itself.

Of course, not only symptomatic and socially harmful patterns have a tendency to stabilize themselves. The same applies to resilient behavior and experience.

Mary

Mary was 20 when I met her. She grew up in a social hot-spot in a high-rise estate in Hamburg. Both her parents were alcoholics. There was a lot of shouting in her family. Her father regularly beat her. After primary school, she went to a special school. The teacher there said to her: "You don't belong in a special school. I'll talk to your parents about you going to the main school." Because her parents didn't care where their daughter went to school, the teacher organized the change. In the main school, Mary was the best in her class. "You should go to the secondary school," suggested one of her teachers. Mary went to the secondary school. She completed her secondary education there and decided to attend the upper level at the grammar school. During this time, she went to the youth welfare office. She explained her situation at home to a social worker and asked how she could move out so that her parents would still be financially responsible for her, but would not know her whereabouts. The social worker organized a place for her in a residential group for young adults and arranged for contact opportunities for both sides via the youth welfare office. After graduating from high school, Mary decided to study sociology and political science. She was an excellent student and completed internships at some of the most renowned research institutions in her field. When her father refused to continue paying for her studies unless she told him her whereabouts, she sued him, successfully. She applied for a scholarship and moved with her boyfriend to Paris, where she continued her studies at the Sorbonne. Then I lost sight of Mary.

Ten years later I thought of her. I considered: The patterns from back then will have continued, in other words: Mary will have continued to use her competencies, with which she moved from misery and poverty ever further towards success. What had become of her? I found her and talked to her on the phone. Dr. Mary So-and-so had become a consultant at the Ministry of This-and-that in Mecklenburg-Vorpommern. Another ten years later I was curious again. By then, Mary was working as a consultant at a federal ministry in Berlin.

What proves itself continues. In ten years I will ask again what Mary is doing.

The story illustrates how biographical sections and life experiences of other people can be used. In therapy, I use the story, for example, to encourage young people who have worked their way out of difficult situations to expect further good developments for themselves. In training and supervision, it can (somewhat as a positive counterpart to "1492") illustrate how psychological and social patterns that have once been established tend to persist throughout life and sometimes across generations. As one can imagine, the story is based on facts, only the name and minor details in the woman's career have been changed.

Stabilizing Therapeutic Successes
Helpful developments are stabilized when they are noticed by the client, when they are accepted as actually having happened and projected permanently into the future. Any interpretation of therapeutic changes aimed at diminishing their significance, for example by portraying the effect as small, uncertain, or only temporary, acts as an internal anti-suggestion that damages the sustainability of the therapeutic results. In therapy, it is important to perceive successes and celebrate them as harbingers of greater successes. It is important to also align therapists to not only focus on problems, but to make every small success of their clients perceptible to them and to celebrate them as signs of a good process.

Celebrating the Garden Bed

My father worked in his garden every day. He loved his garden. One day you would see him pruning the fruit trees, another day he would be building a wooden frame for the pole beans, and then again you would see him digging up a vegetable bed. And in the evening, when the sun was setting, you would see him standing in his garden, looking at his work. If you asked him, "What are you doing?" or "What are you thinking about?" he would say, "I'm looking at what I've done today. I've dug up *all* of this." To work and then celebrate what he had achieved with his work, that was the key to his happiness.

Setting the Next Goal in Sight
For example, when clients qualify positive changes not as "good", but merely as "better", the metaphor of the

horizons lying one behind the other can be used. But it is also important for therapists to not consider the results that clients expect at best as a limit that can only be approached, but as a stage goal, behind which other good goals are waiting. When the clients' goal is reached, we ask them what goal they want to achieve now. Since clients often set their goals far below what can be achieved in a session, it is often necessary to update the clients' goals several times within a session. I would like to pass on this experience to the participants of a therapy training or supervision and invite them to convey a correspondingly confident attitude to their clients.

Behind Every Horizon

When I leave the house and follow the street to the end, I come to a hill with a wide view over the city and the Palatinate Forest. From there I can see the lookout tower on the Humberg on the horizon. If I walk there, I can see the mountains south of the city. If I walk to the next horizon, I see the next horizon and after a few horizons I can already see across to Alsace and the Vosges. Behind every horizon is a next horizon. Behind what now appears to be the best possible, waits what is better and behind that what is even better. You can call what is "better" than the previous state "good", even if we know that it is not yet so good that it could not be even better. Behind every "Good" waits an even "better Good"! It can always be "even better" than it is right now, and if we don't dare to call what is already better "good" now, even though it could be even better, then it is never good for us, and that would actually be a shame. So, let's call it good now and look forward to the even better "Good"!

Protecting One's Own Interests

In supervision, it is important to convey to therapists and other helpers the need to set boundaries in order to protect their own interests or to conserve their own resources, so that they can work in the long term without loss of energy, without resentment or frustration. It can also be important for clients not to live selflessness unconditionally. It seems as if not even the good Lord is completely selfless…

In the Garden of Eden

"I know exactly why the good Lord didn't want Adam and Eve to eat the fruits from his tree," said my father, as he once again stood in the evening light in his garden and looked at a tree full of red apples. "Why?" I asked. "He wanted to eat them himself."

Among the central interests of the therapist are, on the one hand, protection from emotional overload, and on the other hand, the preservation of emotional resonance, i.e., the ability to empathize. I tell the following to some people who are in training and supervision with me, but also to some clients:

On the Same Wavelength

When working as a therapist, it is important to empathize with clients, to resonate with them on a common wavelength, so to speak.

Equally important is not to be swept away by their vibrations. It would be highly unfavorable if the therapist suffers as much as his clients each time. It is already unfavorable if he suffers at all.

In physics class, we learned that two things describe a wave: The frequency of oscillation, which results from the wavelength, and the amplitude, i.e., the deflection or height of the wave.

Please send a nice greeting to your brain: It is welcome to resonate exactly at the frequency of your client, but it does not need to resonate with the same amplitude as the client. On the contrary: The smaller the deflection, i.e., intensity, of your resonance, the less energy you consume, the more joy you have at work, and the more clients you can support. The amplitude of your resonance should be so small that you can work indefinitely and never consume more energy in a day than you have replenished by the next morning.

Adapting the Therapy to the Client—and then Spreading Confidence

A principle of hypnosystemic therapy states: "Not the clients have to fit our methods, but our methods have to fit the clients." Accordingly, Gunther Schmidt, the founder of hypnosystemic work, explains that he is actually not a therapist, but a "reality waiter". The waiter presents the guest with a menu of possibilities, but the guest chooses what suits him (Schmidt 2004, p. 65).

Following Schmidt's work, it is common in hypnosystemic counseling to consistently reinterpret the idea of therapists that the client shows "resistance", a lack of "compliance" or "no insight into the disease" to mean that the clients in question have needs that have not yet been sufficiently considered by the therapist—such as a need for autonomy, belonging to a group other than the therapist's team, recognition of their own worldview, or protection from retraumatization. For therapy to be successful, the client does not necessarily have to adapt to the therapist's offers. It is much more effective if the therapist has the flexibility to adapt to the client's offers.

The Mouse in the Laundry Basket

Once again, my cat has brought a mouse into the house to play with, and once again the mouse has escaped under some cabinet or chair. The cat is long gone in search of new mice, but I have a mouse walking around my apartment. I don't want it to settle in permanently. It can live a happy life outside. For such cases, I have a live trap, a small cage with a door that snaps shut when the mouse goes for the treat inside. I load the trap with cheese and place it next to the sofa where the mouse disappeared. It doesn't take long and the mouse comes out again. Unfortunately, it doesn't go into the trap I set up. Doesn't it like my cheese? I don't know. It takes a different route and jumps into the laundry basket. Not a good place! I'm worried it will chew holes in my clothes. Should I take out the clothes to save them from the mouse? I have a better idea… I carry the basket outside and remove the clothes there, one piece at a time. Last of all, the mouse jumps out, into its freedom.

A Miracle in Stages

Once, a few people came to Jesus who had brought a blind man. "Rabbi, can you heal him?" Jesus looked at the man, licked his finger, and smeared the spit on the man's eyes.

"Open your eyes! What do you see?" he asked the man. The man looked around. "I see people walking around like trees." Then Jesus licked his finger again and smeared spit on the man's eyes again. "What do you see now?" he asked the man. And this time the man saw everything clearly. (Bible according to Martin Luther 2016, Mark 8, 22–25)

I used to think that Jesus' miracles happened in one fell swoop with a "bang" and a "boom". Here I learn that these miracles sometimes took place in a process in several stages. Jesus was not deterred by this. When something started to work, he did more of the same and got more of the same. I'm sure if he had needed three or four or five attempts, he would have taken this time as well. If it's allowed for Jesus, it's okay for us too. Miracles can be a process.

It can also be important not to be deterred by individual failures.

> **No Miracle**
>
> By the way, the thing with miracles didn't always work for Jesus either. If people didn't trust him, it didn't work. Jesus was not deterred and continued—with those who could and wanted to engage with him (Matthew 13:58).
>   If Jesus could afford a few failures, so can we.

In general, all stories that tell of liberation are suitable for therapy.

> **Freeing Birds**
>
> In Cambodia, I saw street vendors selling birds. They did not do this so that the buyers could eat them or keep them as pets. Instead, after paying the purchase price, the customers were allowed to open a small door and release the birds into freedom. Why? Because it brings luck! Certainly to the birds and perhaps to the people as well...

The story can be used, for example, to encourage parents to release their children from a symbiotic or abusive relationship or to honor their start into adult life as a step that brings luck.

It can also be used in other situations where it is about overcoming dependencies or letting go of something that no longer fits into the current phase of life (cf. the liberation of a carp from its bucket, Hammel 2006, p. 74, 2012, p. 70).

References

Bibel nach Martin Luthers Übersetzung (2016) Standardausgabe. Ohne Apokryphen. Bibelgesellschaft, Stuttgart

Hammel S (2006) Der Grashalm in der Wüste. Metaphern und Geschichten in Beratung, Therapie und Seelsorge. impress, Mainz

Hammel S (2012) The blade of grass in the Desert. Storytelling: Forgotten medicine for healing the soul. A story of 100 stories for counselling and therapy. impress, Mainz

Hammel S (2019) Lebensmöglichkeiten entdecken. Veränderung durch therapeutisches Modellieren. Klett-Cotta, Stuttgart

Hammel S (2022) Hypnosystemische Therapie. Das Handbuch für die Praxis. Klett-Cotta, Stuttgart

Hammel S (2024) Transforming lives with hypnosystemic therapy. A practical guide. Routledge, London

Schmidt G (2004) Liebesaffären zwischen Problem und Lösung. Hypnosystemisches Arbeiten in schwierigen Kontexten. Heidelberg, Carl Auer

Zeig J (ed) (1982) Ericksonian approaches to hypnosis and psychotherapy. Brunner, New York

14

Storytelling as a Remedy in Collectively Experienced Crises?

Trailer

This chapter is about the significance of stories for society and the planet. The type of stories told influences the coexistence and self-understanding of nations and peoples. Some narratives promote cooperation and respect, while other stories spread hate and fear. Healing stories of courage, hope, and respect can counteract destructive patterns. Narratives that keep in mind the welfare of the majority and the protection of minorities, and encourage a positive approach to differences, can strengthen the community. To this end, we can share stories that inspire people to take active and powerful action and direct their gaze towards a better future.

"What kind of stories would one have to tell to help the planet?" a seminar participant asked me. "I'm also concerned about that," I replied. "Perhaps the answer becomes a little easier when one asks: Which stories do a people good or not good? I remember how during the Football

World Cup, people from many countries of the world came together in Germany. Everyone was amazed and the whole world talked about how the Germans were different than previously thought. They were imagined to be strict, serious, accurate, and buttoned-up. But the people one encountered were open, cheerful, warm, hospitable, they liked to celebrate and one could easily engage in conversation with them.

Perhaps it's because of this: Months before the event, posters with the motto of the event, 'The world as guests among friends,' were hung in many German cities and especially at the venues of the games. Friendly faces from all over the world were gathered there in harmony, with painted flags on their cheeks. Could it be that it makes a difference if everyone participating in this major event carries this motto 'The world as guests among friends' within them? I notice at least: When the media talks about the refugees of a country with terms like "solidarity", "support", "help" and "welcome culture", the mood is different than when slogans and terms like "The boat is full", "Children instead of Indians", "Asylum abuse" and "Economic refugees" are thrown into the discussion.

It can be observed that nations tell themselves stories about how they came into being and who they therefore are. In France, people tell each other how the French Revolution eliminated the ruling class that had oppressed them. Napoleon is seen as a glorious general. In Germany, people tell each other that the country's role in the First and Second World War gives it a special responsibility for peace in the world. In the USA, people tell each other that the country was founded by pioneers seeking freedom there. Israeli founding stories tell of the persecution of Jews, of Zionist settlers, but also of Moses, to whom the land was promised by God, of the walls of Jericho that fell before the Israeli warriors, and of the glorious King David.

There is often little to no mention of the rulers' bloodshed against minorities in their own country and the subjugated neighboring peoples.

Perhaps it's not bad if the bad is forgotten—because there might be better stories that a people can tell about themselves. However, it would be desirable for the members of the oppressed groups that the stories of the victors paid respect to their families and peoples and allowed justice to be done.

We can tell stories about people from our midst who have dedicated their lives to something good and thus achieved something good.

We can tell each other stories that focus attention on favorable patterns, where values are realized in the attitude of "both-and" instead of in the style of "either-or", where cooperation ("non-zero-sum games") is more in the foreground than those of subjugation and war ("zero-sum games").

We can tell narratives that promote "the greatest possible happiness for the greatest possible number" and at the same time keep an eye on the protection of minorities (Hammel 2022, p. 13; Hammel 2024).

We can tell that "all people are equal" and therefore deserve equal respect and that "all people are different" and therefore deserve individual treatment that addresses their unique situation.

We can tell stories that do not answer bad with bad, but make distinctions between the presumably good or originally "well-intentioned" intentions of people to behave as it used to lead to an experience of belonging, protection, and autonomy—although the implementation strategies for this are now often unsuitable, self-damaging and socially harmful.

We can tell whatever has led us and others from an experience of passive suffering into shaping, everything that has brought us from experiences of being driven into powerful action and has led us from the area of limited choices in thinking and acting into the area of greater choices. Stories that deal with opportunities and possibilities and all stories that widen the view and the heart—towards other people and other living beings, to other times and spaces and other possibilities of life—we can put in the center of that public that hears our word and carries it on.

That stories are a remedy for a humanity that has become entangled in destructive patterns, I have no doubt. The challenge is to bring narratives of courage and hope and respect for the otherness of the other to the people, despite all the hate and fear stories that have been circulated. I see it as our task to do that wherever possible.

References

Hammel S (2022) Hypnosystemische Therapie. Das Handbuch für die Praxis. Klett-Cotta, Stuttgart

Hammel S (2024) Transforming lives with hypnosystemic therapy. A practical guide. Routledge, London

Appendix: Therapy and Further Education Opportunities

> This section provides information on how to find therapists
> who use stories in therapy in the way presented here, as
> well as how to further educate oneself as a coach, consult-
> ant, therapist, or counselor in this field.

Those seeking therapy, coaching, or supervision with therapeutic storytelling as an integrated working method can
find out from the author (www.stefanhammel.de) which
therapists work in a similar way as presented here. In addition to physical meetings on site, therapeutic sessions in
video format should also be considered. Experience has
shown that working with video sessions is just as effective
as sessions in physical presence.

S. Hammel, *Learning Therapeutic Storytelling*,
https://doi.org/10.1007/978-3-662-69110-6

Seminars and training opportunities for therapeutic storytelling are:

1. Institute for Hypnosystemic Consultation, Kaiserslautern, physically or online
(Stefan Hammel)
Seminars (12 days) as part of the "Hypnosystemic Therapy" training (also bookable separately, with individual seminars in English available at www.stefanhammel.com)
www.hsb-westpfalz.de

2. Institute for Culture and Religion, Berlin, physically
(Jean-Otto Domanski)
Seminars (6 days) as part of the hypnosystemic pastoral care training "Words that work" (also bookable separately).
www.inkur-berlin.de

GPSR Compliance

The European Union's (EU) General Product Safety Regulation (GPSR) is a set of rules that requires consumer products to be safe and our obligations to ensure this.

If you have any concerns about our products, you can contact us on ProductSafety@springernature.com

In case Publisher is established outside the EU, the EU authorized representative is:

Springer Nature Customer Service Center GmbH
Europaplatz 3
69115 Heidelberg, Germany

The manufacturer's authorised representative in the EU is Springer
Nature Customer Service Centre GmbH, Europaplatz 3, 69115 Heidelberg,
Germany. If you have any concerns regarding our products, please
contact ProductSafety@springernature.com

Printed and bound by CPI Group (UK) Ltd, Croydon, CR0 4YY
24/04/2026
02096358-0001